Full Figure
Fitness

A Program for
Teaching Overweight Adults

Bonnie D. Kingsbury
Bethesda Hospital

Life Enhancement Publications
Champaign, Illinois

Library of Congress Cataloging-in-Publication Data

Kingsbury, Bonnie D., 1948–
    Full figure fitness : a program for teaching overweight adults / Bonnie D.
Kingsbury.
        p.   cm.
    Bibliography: p.
    Includes index.
    ISBN 0-87322-923-1
    1. Reducing exercises. 2. Obesity—Exercise therapy.   I. Title.
RA781.6.K56 1988
613.7′1—dc19   87-31673
                                                          CIP

Developmental Editor: Sue Wilmoth, PhD
Production Director: Ernie Noa
Projects Manager: Lezli Harris
Copy Editor: Lise Rodgers
Assistant Editor: Julie Anderson
Typesetters: Theresa Bear and Sonnie Bowman
Text Design: Keith Blomberg
Text Layout: Denise Mueller
Photographs by Eastgate Photographers
Artwork by Century Printing
Special thanks to exercise models Nancy Black, Carol Hockensmith, and Nancy J. Karlen
Editorial consultant: Corey Lincoln
Content advisor: Debra A. Knight, MS, ATC and Orland W. Wooley, PhD
Printed By: United Graphics

ISBN: 0-87322-923-1

Printed in the United States of America

10 9 8 7 6 5 4 3 2 1

Life Enhancement Publications
A Division of Human Kinetics Publishers, Inc.
Box 5076, Champaign, IL 61820
1-800-342-5457
1-800-334-3665 (in Illinois)

Dedication

To my original Full Figure Fitness participants,
without whose candor and support my dream
might have remained in Fantasyland.

To me it's inconceivable
That one could find believable
The prospect one must have a shape
Exactly like his chum.
I simply won't apologize
For being of a grander size—
When everyone's a seedless grape
It's great to be a plum.

Victor Buono
From: *It Could Be Verse*

Acknowledgments

Few of us have an opportunity to put our experience in writing. Those of us who have this opportunity realize that it takes more than an author and a keyboard to complete the effort. Without the support of family, friends, and professional guidance to get the job done, far fewer books would ever be written.

I wish to thank, first of all, my husband, Steve, for his loving assistance, and my children, Brent and Bridget for their uncomplaining patience while mom typed 'just one more page.' Without the support of each of them, this project would have been almost impossible.

I am especially grateful to Dr. Sue Wilmoth of Human Kinetics Publishers for her faith in me and her confidence in Full Figure Fitness. Thanks to Dr. Linda Hall of the Christ Hospital for directing me to Human Kinetics. Special thanks to Dr. Wayne Wooley for his excellent research material as well as his enthusiasm for the book.

I also wish to express my appreciation to Dick Jones of the YMCA of the USA for his encouragement in 'taking my show on the road.' Thanks also to Sue Regnier for her direction and organizational efforts. And last, never least, I'd like to thank my friends and former colleagues at the Clermont County YMCA for backing me every inch of the way.

Contents

Preface

Another fitness program? Isn't the market saturated?

Indeed, many of us have a variety of fitness classes at our disposal. Weight training programs, water exercise, and aerobics classes are all available to help us get into shape while enjoying the company of others in the same predicament. But how many of us would participate in an exercise class on an ongoing basis if we found the experience overwhelming or humiliating?

This book is about a different kind of fitness program—one that is geared to people who are more in need of exercise than most of us, but who are less likely to take advantage of standard exercise programs. You'll learn about the people for whom these special classes are designed, why they need a different kind of program, what kinds of problems they encounter, and how to become sensitive and responsive to their needs.

I became aware of the need for a special exercise program for overweight adults while I was teaching a fitness class a few years ago. Usually the programs attracted men and women of average weight and varying levels of aerobic conditioning. There were always several overweight people in the early weeks of each new session. They had more difficulty keeping up with the pace of the program, and their progress was relatively slow. Often toward the end of an eight-week session only one or two of them were still attending. I admired the tenacity of these few, but I also realized that a change in format was needed that would allow overweight people to exercise in a less intimidating environment.

The concept of *Full Figure Fitness* was inspired by a conversation I overheard in the locker room. Two women were discussing their efforts to tone up. Over the din of running water and the whirring of hair dryers I heard one shout to the other, "What they really ought to give us is an exercise class for fat ladies." They snickered, and I went to work.

It will be important for anyone planning to conduct a Full Figure Fitness class to read this book in its entirety. The FFF program is based on much research and experience. All of the material contained herein is useful and relevant. The instructor need not become an expert in obesity, but a general understanding of its causes and effects, along with a thorough knowledge of sensible exercise guidelines, will expand her ability to address the needs of her students.

By reading the manual and following its guidelines, you will learn about how you can offer a quality exercise program to overweight and obese individuals; what practical advice experts have to offer in the fields of psychology, eating disorders, physical therapy, and nutrition; what the most up-to-date theories are regarding the causes and complex nature of obesity; how you can successfully market and promote the program; and what exercise techniques are most appropriate for an overweight population.

Developing the Full Figure Fitness program has opened my eyes to the problems of being a fat person in a diet-conscious country where appearance is often the precursor of acceptance. I have seen again and again the positive effect this program has on its participants. For many it has laid the foundation for developing healthier lifestyles and improved outlooks on life. A good example is a former student of mine who approached me after our workout one wet, dreary April morning. A smile graced her face as she gazed out the window. "I'll tell you something, Bonnie," she said leaning against the wall and studying the dampness outside. "If it hadn't been for this Full Figure class, on a morning like this I'd usually be staring out my kitchen window, stuffin' my face, and feelin' like hell."

Bonnie D. Kingsbury

Chapter
1
The Whys and Wherefores of Full Figure Fitness

This book is for fitness educators and health care providers who understand that fitness goals will vary from person to person. A runner may not consider himself truly fit until he can run a mile in under six minutes, while a fat person may be thrilled with his fitness when he is able to walk around the block without becoming exhausted. We do not all have the same capabilities, objectives, or motivations. For those of us hoping to improve our physical condition, our methods should correspond to both our abilities and our limitations.

Full Figure Fitness (FFF) is an exercise program whose time has come. In this country overweight adults represent more than 35% of the population, and their numbers are growing. Yet society's attitude toward obesity is contemptuous and critical. Overweight people are ostracized and made to feel guilty. Their desire to fit in supports a $15-billion-a-year diet industry, which holds out promises it can't possibly keep.

FFF offers what overweight people need: not rigid diets and negative attitudes, but a comprehensive program of fitness in the company of others who share similar concerns. The program doesn't make judgments or encourage unattainable goals. It simply recognizes the special need for this population to receive health education and a schedule of regular exercise. A sensitive, sound exercise program can give many people the incentive they need to pursue healthy lifestyle changes.

Americans: Fitness or Fatness?

In the past decade much attention has been focused on American fitness and health. We are exposed to a great deal of information and advertising that might lead us to believe most Americans have adopted healthy lifestyles of regular exercise and nutritious eating. Television commercials and newspaper and magazine ads depict slim, attractive men and women engaging in vigorous activity, eating nourishing foods, and generally epitomizing "the good life."

But take a look around. Where *are* all these lean, active people? Though it is certainly true that more people are exercising today than a generation ago, it is also true that American "fatness" far exceeds American fitness. Visit your local shopping center or supermarket, and you will probably get a pretty realistic picture of the shape we're in. The problem has also affected 25% of our children. If advertisers were to depict things as they really are, we would be more likely to see ads that feature an overweight family, recumbent in front of the TV set, nibbling on junk food.

Most of us aren't perfectly proportioned, nor are we even in very good physical condition. There is a great number of people who, for a variety of reasons, are fat. And they are usually not happy about it. Some are willing to try anything to reduce their weight, and they wage a constant battle to control it. But once a person's weight has fluctuated over a period of time, keeping the pounds off becomes increasingly difficult. Rigid dieting produces only temporary results. Moreover, dieting can produce severe frustration and depression. Everybody's got to eat, and constant fretting over every mouthful is a drain on one's well-being.

The issue of overweight needs to be addressed realistically. Exercise is a favorable alternative to strict dieting because its benefits include more than just weight loss. Exercise also tends to help people focus attention on other healthful habits as their activity increases.

But many overweight people avoid exercise because it is difficult and tedious, and because, in a group setting (which is the preferred method of exercising for many), it can be embarrassing. Just as advertising companies promote fitness as a beauty aid, fitness programs also seem to be directed toward a very slim group of people. Overweight Americans are not properly represented in exercise classes. And because their numbers are ever-increasing, it seems reasonable that they should receive a personalized fitness program that considers their particular wants, needs, and abilities.

Overview: The Program in Brief

Full Figure Fitness was designed to serve the fitness and health needs of overweight and obese[1] individuals. Through a comprehensive program of exercise, education, and camaraderie, its goals include the following:

- To encourage positive lifestyle changes through regular exercise and realistic goal-setting.
- To deliver the message that fat people can become fit people, or at least *more* fit. Many obese adults think they are too fat to participate in an exercise program. They often attempt to lose weight without increasing physical activity. As most of you know, such efforts are usually counterproductive. Under professional supervision, a well-planned, comprehensive, and enjoyable exercise program can be started at any time. The main objective should be enhanced fitness, not weight loss.
- To reach out to a large number of people who have become segregated from the social mainstream. Overweight men and women prefer to exercise in a nonthreatening atmosphere that leaves them free to work at their own pace.
- To instill in the participants a sense of personal responsibility for their health. There is no magic formula for achieving a sound body; it requires effort and discipline. Instructors can guide and encourage their students, but lasting responsibility lies with the individual.
- To offer a sound exercise program based on safe progression and the special needs of overweight exercisers. Until now overweight men and women had little motivation to affiliate with wellness programs or fitness facilities on a long-term basis. After several weeks of uncomfortable, embarrassing attempts at exercising with a group, they often drop out. Let's face it: A 200-pound woman attempting to follow a Jane Fonda type lead probably won't hold out for the duration.

---

[1]According to the experts, *overweight* means that one weighs more than 10 percent above his or her "ideal" weight when compared to age, height, sex, and body frame as indicated on standard insurance tables. A muscular person can be overweight without having excess body fat. *Overfat* means that a person has excess body fat. A person of "normal" weight could be overfat. *Obese* refers to a condition exceeding 20 percent of an individual's average or recommended weight. Though these three terms are different by definition, they will be used interchangeably as a matter of convenience.

FFF will help students improve their physical condition without making them feel out of sync with the class. The FFF program addresses the physical capabilities of overweight students at all levels of fitness. Beginners' exercises are manageable for beginners, and more advanced exercises are challenging for ardent enthusiasts. The Full Figure Fitness plan inspires its participants to join with others who enjoy the benefits of healthy, active lifestyles.

The Instructor's Role

The FFF instructor is the mainstay of the program. Because the program makes an important statement about the rights of the overweight, many eyes will be on the instructor to see if this FFF philosophy is indeed valid. A poor or inexperienced instructor can get the program off to a bad start, which could result in a quick finish.

FFF is not a conventional fitness program. A lean body, which is often a high priority for many of us who decide to exercise, is not emphasized in this program because it is not a realistic goal. Most participants will tone up, lose inches, improve aerobic capacity, and feel better after the completion of the first session. But they will not alter their body composition appreciably through exercise alone. The instructor must, therefore, be flexible in her willingness to modify different programs to suit different needs. If she teaches other exercise programs, she has probably experienced more observable changes in the participants than she will in FFF. In

FFF she will discover the changes to be more subtle, though equally (if not more) significant.

The FFF instructor should be an experienced, achievement-oriented leader who enjoys a challenge. She should be an informed educator, a terrific listener, and once in a while, even a stand-up comic. She will work hard to motivate her classes to exert themselves from the start; and she will need to continuously sell them on fitness to keep them going. Helping students get from point *A* to point *B* requires the skill of a true professional.

Some participants will join the program expecting miracles; others won't know what to expect; still others will have realistic goals in mind. The instructor will have to deliver a well-balanced exercise program in which participants augment both their physical conditioning and their understanding of fitness. But what the fitness leader sows in hard work she will reap in the joys of accomplishment and the appreciation of those she teaches.

The format of FFF is more informal and less restricted than many others—it is intended to be chattier and more relaxed. Its members enjoy, and often need, the opportunity for socialization with their peers. An outlet for pent-up hostility is important. If a teacher has become accustomed to conducting a highly structured program of a style similar to military boot camp, he or she is probably *not* a good candidate to lead Full Figure Fitness.

This book will help you start developing your own program of fitness for overweight adults. But in order to maximize its potential for success, it will be necessary for the fitness leader to keep abreast of the current information available in the areas of exercise and overweight.

Chapter
2
Understanding the Full Figure Participant

Much of the scientific and lay literature today emphasizes the numerous risks of being overweight. On the whole, it paints a rather bleak picture for men and women who carry more body fat than is necessary for survival. Instructors should acquaint themselves with material that treats the problem of obesity on an objective level. The more familiar you become with the information available on this topic, the more effective will be your leadership both in and out of the classroom.

My own research has given me new insights into the most appropriate teaching methods for this population. Had I begun teaching FFF using nothing but my instincts to guide me, the program might have had an abrupt ending.

Let me give you an example. Before completing plans for the program, I had intended to perform a body composition analysis on each FFF member. I mistakenly assumed that measurable changes in body fat would occur within months of participating in Full Figure Fitness. But after researching data concerning physiological changes in overweight people who exercise, I understood that pre- and postskinfold analyses might be unwise; many of these people would not show a substantial increase in lean body mass. If I'd carried

out my original plan, students who showed no appreciable change in their body fat after a period of regular exercise might have become disappointed in themselves and in the FFF program.

I am sure that my readers are aware of the derogatory information regarding fat. In an industry based on the idea that a lean body is a healthier body, the very word *fat* sends us running for cover. The following chapters may contain information contrary to your understanding of overweight. I wish to present the reader with a slightly different perspective on the subject of moderate, stable overweight.

Profile of the Full Figure Participant

The typical student in this program is 35 years old and female. She is moderately overweight (between 10 and 20 percent over her target weight) and has tried every diet in the book. In fact, she could talk circles around most of us when it comes to calorie counting and nutrition information. She is intelligent, articulate, and has a quick wit and a well-developed sense of humor.

In spite of her ready smile, our average student describes feeling stressed and in need of an outlet for her tension. In most conventional exercise classes I've taught, students haven't been quite so candid about personal problems. Perhaps the difference between FFF participants and these others can be explained by the fact that FFFers tend to have more medical problems and so often spend more time discussing their medical histories with the instructor than do students in conventional fitness programs.

Under these circumstances, the FFF participant may consider her candor regarding stress appropriate. Her willingness to share her frustrations in welcome surroundings where she is unencumbered by criticism and judgment may hasten improvements both physically and emotionally.

Society's aversion to anything outside the norm has had a profound effect on people who are overweight. I'll never forget the day one of my students asked for additional exercises she could do at home. I recommended that she take walks around the neighborhood. Her response to what I considered pretty basic advice brought home to me the injustices dealt to the obese. "Oh, no way!" she protested, flinging up her arms as if warding off an attacker. "You couldn't possibly know what it feels like to go for a walk and have kids holler out a passing car, 'Hey, check out the lardass!' and things like that." Imagine what it must be like to cope with that kind of prejudice day after day!

The average FFF participant is inquisitive about exercise and insightful about how it feels to be fat in a society that repudiates obesity. Yet despite adversities, her remarkable wit and convulsive laughter often generate their own cardiovascular workouts. Sometimes it's confusing as to which is more exhausting—the exercises or the guffaws! Of the many fitness and wellness programs I have taught, Full Figure Fitness will always be the most meaningful. The warm, supportive atmosphere generated by my students has given me the insight, understanding, and determination to make this program succeed.

Societal Attitudes Toward Fat People

Being fat is considered socially unacceptable. Fat people are treated as objects of ridicule and con-

tempt. They suffer bias in education, employment, social life, and even medical treatment. One of my students offered a telling example of the pressures fat people are under to conform to difficult and arbitrary demands. She had scheduled an appointment with a physician for treatment of nothing more than a lingering viral infection, nonetheless, the doctor's opening words to her were, "Well, I think the first thing we should talk about is how you're going to take off about fifty pounds"!

Repeated studies have demonstrated that cultural attitudes toward body types are commonly shared, independent of an individual's own size. In several studies (Lerner & Korn, 1972; Lerner & Schroeder, 1971; Staffieri, 1967) subjects who were asked to describe pictures of endomorphs (round body types) typically used the words *lazy, mean,* and *dirty*; descriptions of mesomorphs (muscular body types) included the words *strong, healthy,* and *brave*; ectomorphs (thin body types) were also described negatively, but not to the same degree as endomorphs (see Figure 2.1). Interestingly, in each study, subjects gave similar descriptions of body types regardless of their own size—fat people said negative things about fat bodies, muscular people said positive things about muscular bodies, and so on.

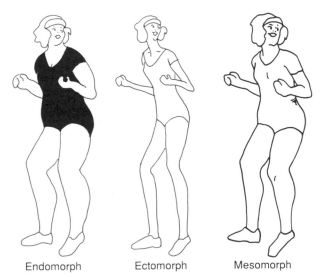

Endomorph   Ectomorph   Mesomorph

Figure 2.1 Three basic body builds.

There is also evidence that bias against fat begins in early childhood. In one experiment (Richardson, Goodman, Hastorf, & Dornbusch, 1961), children were shown pictures of normal, thin, and fat children, as well as children with disabilities. The fat children were selected as the most unattractive and unpopular.

In her book *Eating Disorders*, author and researcher Hilde Bruch says of the plight of the obese,

> There is a great deal of talk about the weakness and self-indulgence of overweight people who eat too much. Very little is said about the self-ishness and self-indulgence involved in a life which makes one's appearance the center of all values.

Society's rejection of obesity is exemplified, among other things, by the design of public accommodations. Seats in airplanes, theaters, and restaurants are often too narrow or small to accommodate large bodies. Certain foreign and American sports cars cater to a thin population by making front seat space so confined that a big body couldn't even get into the vehicle, let alone sit comfortably inside.

The health industry often blames rising health costs on overweight Americans' gluttonous lifestyles. Blue Cross runs an ad depicting an overweight man with bulging stomach and straining shirt buttons captioned: "One of the reasons for the high cost of health care." Beneath the illustration is a graph indicating the rising costs of coronary care units. The implication is, of course, that obesity causes heart attacks, and is therefore responsible for high health costs. However, scientific evidence indicates that obesity is not always a primary cause of heart attacks. Inactivity, stress, frequent weight fluctuations, heredity, and poor nutritional habits are among the major contributors to coronary disease. Furthermore, increased coronary care costs are also due to expensive, high-tech medical equipment and to the profit margins of the health industry.

Members of the National Association to Aid Fat Americans (NAAFA), as well as volumes of scientific evidence, stress that being fat does not result solely from lack of willpower: Body type, childhood habits, heredity, and metabolism also contribute to obesity. (This topic will be discussed further under "Determinants of Obesity" in this chapter.) NAAFA argues that fat people feel isolated because they are socially excluded, and that an individual should not have to be thin to enjoy acceptance by others. Furthermore, there are very few effective treatments for obesity. As one expert put it, *If "cure" from obesity is defined as reduction to ideal weight and maintenance of that weight for five years, a person is more likely to recover from almost any form of cancer than from obesity* (Greenwood, 1983, p. 40).

Fat as a Feminine Problem

Women are stigmatized by obesity more than men. Clients of diet centers, eating disorder clinics, and nutritional services are overwhelmingly female, as are the members of FFF. Research shows that the price paid for having an "unacceptable" body is not just psychological or emotional. Obesity and overweight may actually be preventing many intelligent, capable women from pursuing careers for which they are otherwise well suited.

A study (Goldblatt, Moore, & Stunkard, 1965) of 1,660 adult residents of midtown Manhattan demonstrated that, compared with nonobese women, obese women are less likely to rise above, and more likely to fall below, the socioeconomic status of their parents. No such correlation was found among the men studied. The researchers also reported that, although the percentage of thin men is the same for all three social classes (10 percent for lower, 9 percent for middle, and 12 percent for upper class), the percentage of thin women is directly proportional to social class (9 percent, 19 percent, and 37 percent respectively). The authors state:

> In the midtown Manhattan society we do not have to look far to see the image of the slim, attractive female as portrayed throughout the popular culture. . . . A selection process may operate so that in any status-conferring situation, such as a promotion at work or marriage to a higher status male, thinner women may be preferentially selected over their competitors. (pp. 1042–1043)

In a study of 1964 graduates of a large middle-class suburban high school, Canning and Mayer (1966) found that although obese and nonobese girls did not differ on objective measures of intellectual ability or in the percentage who applied for college admission, 51.9 percent of the nonobese high school girls went to college the year after graduation, while only 31.6 percent of the obese girls did. The corresponding figures for boys show no statistically significant difference: 53.3 percent of the nonobese and 49.9 percent of the obese high school graduates went to college.

The researchers state:

> If obese adolescents have difficulty in attending college, a substantial proportion may experience a drop in social class, or fail to advance beyond present levels. Education, occupation, and income are social-class variables

that are strongly interrelated. A vicious circle, therefore, may begin as a result of college admission discrimination, preventing the obese from rising in the social-class system. (p. 1174)

On the basis of these two studies, W.J. Cahnman (1968) concluded that "obesity, especially as far as girls are concerned, is not so much a mark of low socioeconomic status as a condemnation to it" (p. 290).

Anthropologist Anne Scott Beller (1978) writes,

the ideal of feminine beauty has thus come increasingly within the span of the past half century, to reflect a male ideal model in preference to a typically female one. . . . People tend to ape their betters, and women's aspirations to the unmodulated physiques of men express unvoiced, and until recently, probably largely unconscious, judgments about the nature of male status and privilege as compared to their own. But from an anthropometric point of view, the trend is a dubious one: female fleshiness is a fact of biological life, and one that has every appearance of having been programmed into the species long ago by nature. (pp. 57–58)

Determinants of Obesity

Overweight is not always a simple matter of taking in more calories than are burned off. The law of thermodynamics, which states that energy output equals energy input, may not be the only causal factor in obesity. Several conditions (discussed later in this chapter) may determine why certain bodies more readily store and more reluctantly deplete extra fat.

Although there are many causes of obesity, I will examine only those most common to members of FFF. I have omitted the subject of overeating per se because its relationship to obesity is obvious and requires no additional insight. However, the reader should appreciate that *overeating is as often a symptom of obesity as it is a cause.*

Heredity

Ancestry is a major determinant of body size and shape. Claude Bouchard of Quebec's Laval University has studied body weight within families. His findings show that adopted children are more like their biological parents than their adoptive parents in distribution of body fat and in size of fat cells. Researchers can predict obesity based on hereditary predisposition. The probability of obesity in adulthood is 80 percent for adolescents having two obese parents, 40 percent for adolescents having one obese parent, and 10 percent for adolescents with two normal-weight parents.

The Fat Cell Theory

In 1967, Dr. Jules Hirsch of New York's Rockefeller University introduced evidence that there are two kinds of obesity. In one kind, known as hyperplastic obesity, there are too many fat cells. In the second type, called hypertrophic obesity, there exists the normal number of cells, but they each contain too much fat. Dr. Hirsch contends that in the latter type of obesity, normal weight is easier to reach and sustain because, with weight loss, the cells will shrink markedly. In hyperplastic obesity, however, all those extra fat cells work very hard to retain their stores, and weight is gained readily and lost with difficulty.

Dr. Hirsch further demonstrated that the number of fat cells (adipocytes) increases most during the times when the body is growing fastest: during the last few weeks before birth, during the first two years of life, and during puberty. After puberty the number of fat cells does not appear to increase appreciably (except during periods of rapid weight gain or at levels above 60 percent of normal weight). Rather, the existing cells expand to hold more fat. For women, pregnancy may be another time of fat cell growth (see "Pregnancy and Permanent Weight Gain" in this chapter).

Heredity also determines the distribution of fat in bodies. Obesity specialists recognize two overweight body types: "apples" (mostly men) who carry more weight in the upper torso and abdomen; and "pears" (mostly women) who develop excess fat in the hips, thighs, and buttocks. Fat that is distributed below the abdomen is more stable, and therefore more difficult to get rid of (this is certainly no revelation to my female readers! Instructors who lead co-ed classes will observe that the male participants typically lose weight much more readily through exercise than the females); however, fat distributed in the upper torso and abdomen places a greater burden on the organs and cardiovascular system, and is therefore a greater threat to health.

Environment—The Development of Nutritional Habits

Cultural differences can affect a person's dietary habits and weight. The American diet is high in fat and sugar and low in fiber. Americans have a high incidence of obesity. Countries such as China and Japan have diets that are rich in fiber and low in fat, and consequently have a lower incidence of obesity.

Parents can instill poor eating habits in their children. Our hurried lifestyles promote fewer planned meals that include the four basic food groups. Instead, we have become attracted to fast foods, which are seldom as nutritious as they are convenient. Without proper guidance, children will eat excessive amounts of high sugar and fattening treats, which leads to the production and storage of extra body fat.

During preadolescence, prevention of obesity is more successful than its treatment. As I have mentioned, evidence suggests that overeating during this period causes an increase in the number of fat cells (adipocyte hyperplasia), thus increasing the possibility of obesity. Since lifestyle habits begin early, the sooner healthful controls are developed, the better.

Pregnancy and Permanent Weight Gain

This section will be especially appreciated by the many women who remain steadfast in their belief that they never had a weight problem until they had kids!

In her book, *Fat and Thin: A Natural History of Obesity* (1977), Anne Scott Beller discusses "the relationship between the mother's food intake during pregnancy and the developmental and nutritional status of the newborn baby at birth . . . as two sides of the same coin" (p. 82). Since the developing fetus lives solely on blood sugar, or glucose, the regulation of glucose levels in the mother's blood is critical. During pregnancy the fetus is also dependent on the mother's supply of insulin until shortly before birth. Insulin is the hormone secreted by the pancreas that keeps blood sugar at a constant level in the circulating blood.

As fetal demands for blood sugar rise, the mother's insulin output increases. Excess insulin can cause increased fat storage in the mother, as insulin acts directly on fat cell membranes, binding them in a way that prevents fat from escaping back into the bloodstream. Insulin tries to insure

that all the fat it rounds up remains in storage. Most overweight people have excessive insulin because their cells seem to be resistant to it and their bodies produce more insulin to overcome this resistance.

If the mother's fat cells become resistant to the insulin, her pancreas will produce increasing amounts of it. Her insulin levels will increase, and more food will be converted and stored as fat. If this overproduction response does not dissipate after birth, there will be problems of weight gain. Beller states that

> from now on, every time the new mother eats a meal containing carbohydrates and sugar, and thus flooding her circulating blood with glucose, the beta cells of her pancreas will respond on cue to secreting their by now predictable surplus of insulin . . . her glucose level will fall in response to the oversupply of insulin, and she will feel hungry well before her nutritional status gives her any reason to. (p. 83)

Unless such a person strictly controls her diet, she runs the risk of substantial weight gain.

Further research will be necessary before definitive statements can be made regarding the relationship between pregnancy and obesity, but at this time it appears likely that there is a correlation in some cases.

Refined Carbohydrates: Revenge of the Twinkies

Based on my own experience with overweight people and how they got that way, both inactivity and addiction to sweets seem to be the predominant predicaments of FFF students. Many's the morning I've spotted one of my students munching on a candy bar or sipping a soft drink (or both) before class. I always issue a brief and friendly reminder about the hazards of junk food. I'm not imparting any great wisdom—my students are perfectly aware that junk food is not good for them. But I remain hopeful that eventually my gentle nagging will make an impression. If not, I am comfortable in the knowledge that I have discussed this timely topic in my classes. As informed adults, each of us must ultimately assume responsibility for our own choices in life.

Research has documented time and again the damaging effects of refined carbohydrates, particularly sugar. The refining processes concentrate sugar up to eight times as much as they do flour. Eating excessive amounts of refined sugar products can therefore quite clearly cause problems that lead to obesity.

Most food gets into the bloodstream in the form of sugar. The hormone insulin, as previously mentioned, responds to the blood levels of sugar, or glucose, which is the only type of sugar that circulates through the bloodstream. The amount of glucose in the blood depends on what, when, and how much has been eaten. When we eat, our glucose level rises. If we've eaten a meal rich in processed sugars, our glucose level will become even higher.

When the blood sugar level gets too high, the body lowers it by releasing insulin from the pancreas into the bloodstream. The faster the blood sugar level rises, the more intense the reaction of the pancreas, resulting in too much insulin pouring into the bloodstream. Ironically, when we eat or drink too much processed sugar, our blood sugar levels change from too high to too low, a condition known as rebound hypoglycemia. (Remember that we are talking here about concentrated, refined, or processed sugar, not natural sugar, such as that found in fruit.)

As a result of repeated cycles of overindulging in "goodies," we begin to exhibit the classic symptoms of low blood sugar (hypoglycemia or hyperinsulinism)—headaches, fatigue, tension, and depression. At these times the obese person often feels desperately hungry for the very food that got him in this mess in the first place—sugar. Thus sugar is used to relieve the problem it caused, and the cycle of addiction begins again.

In their book, *Stop Dieting Because Dieting Makes You Fat* (1985), Cannon and Einzig state,

> Processed sugars make you fat for three reasons. First, they contain no nourishment and therefore cheat the body's natural desire for nourishment. Second, because they are concentrated and heavy in calories, they deceive the appetite. . . . Third, and most important, processed sugars make you fat because they disturb the insulin hormone. Processed sugars are the link between obesity, diabetes, and heart disease.

I'd like to tape that quotation to the snack and soda machines in many buildings, but I don't think it would prevent all those quarters from clanging to their destinations. I've stood by in amazement as little children become violent when denied use of the candy or pop machine. Often an embarrassed and exasperated mother will relent and hand over the necessary coins to pacify the hysterical little. . .tyke (who would have been better off without the reinforcements).

America's overuse of refined sugar and white flour should be a concern for all health and fitness educators. Despite society's purported new awareness of fitness concerns, adults and children in this country are becoming fatter and fatter and less inclined to expend energy. We should be alerted to the dangers of unbalanced diets and passive lifestyles. As fitness educators we must strive to develop in our students a sense of personal responsibility for their health and well-being and that of their children, as well as accountability for their actions.

How Stress Can Promote Overweight

Emotions can play a role in obesity in that frustration in one area may lead to excessive gratification in another. (The fact that obesity is more prevalent in lower socioeconomic levels is a case in point.) A 1981 study by University of Cincinnati psychologists Orland and Susan Wooley proposes two hypotheses in the relationship of stress to overeating. The first holds that "long standing dissatisfaction may result in compensatory overeating. Sources of dissatisfaction may include environmental stressors, deprivation of other biological needs, or chronic states such as anxiety and depression" (p. 55). The second hypothesis states that "eating or overeating is an immediate response to acute distress" (p. 55). The Wooleys admit, however, that both hypotheses are difficult to test, and that more information is needed for a definite conclusion. They further suggest that people who have weight problems often develop eating disorders from constantly worrying about food.

Based on clinical studies of obese patients, W.W. Hamburger (1951) proposed that overeating occurs as a response to nonspecific tensions; as a substitute gratification when other areas of life provide few satisfactions; as a response to underlying emotional illness; and as an addictive phenomenon in which food is used to produce sedation by virtue of its previous associations with a sense of well-being and security.

In one of the first attempts to categorize disordered eating patterns associated with obesity, A.J. Stunkard (1959) described the syndromes of night eating and binge eating, both of which he considers related to life stresses. (Night eating seems to be a more common occurrence in FFF students than binge eating. As readers well know, food ingested late at night is destined for storage.)

Studies on binge eating strongly suggest a relationship between overeating and stress. Periods of binge eating are often precipitated by a stressful event. Binge eating is also associated with self-condemnation. Several FFF students have confirmed these findings. They concur that their binges almost always follow a bad experience. One woman stated the problem this way: "When I'm stuffing down one cookie after another, I don't really taste any of it. When I eat like that, I'm hungry all right, but not for food. Anytime I'm really upset, I just pig out and don't think about it."

Compulsive eating may also be used as an anesthetic to deaden feelings. Author Susie Orbach (1978) states that "all negative feelings get harnessed to complaints and self-loathing about body size and eating habits and the fat provides a less threatening issue to worry about than other possible problems" (p. 47). Fat may also be used as a conscious or unconscious protection from feelings of competitiveness. It may keep the person out of competition altogether, or it may be used as an attempt to mask feelings of competitiveness.

Orbach also discusses fat as a rebellion against the powerlessness of a woman, against social pressure to look and act in a certain way in order to fulfill an externally imposed image of what is acceptable. She says,

> for many women, compulsive eating and being fat have become one way to avoid being marketed or seen as the ideal woman: 'My fat says . . . take me for who I am, not for who I'm supposed to be. If you are really interested in me, you can wade through the layers and find out who I am.' (p. 9)

Dieting—Credibility or Corpulence?

It is paradoxical but true that the "cure" for the problem of overweight may be worse than the problem itself. Our national obsession and the $15-billion-dollar-a-year industry that supports it may be, in reality, a metabolic fat mill.

Americans spend a fortune on appetite suppressants (even though appetite often isn't the main reason for overeating). Our society congratulates anyone on a diet. Dieting affords instant acceptance

and credibility. Diet books are often best-sellers, regardless of their creator's credentials.

In a 1982 editorial entitled "The Beverly Hills Eating Disorder . . ." psychologists Wooley and Wooley describe *The Beverly Hills Diet* as "targeting anorexics." The book was written by a woman who lost over seventy pounds on a diet of little more than mangoes and watermelon. Its author, Judy Mazel, discusses her favorite method of responding to food binges: The day after a binge she recommends eating loads of fruit, "which creates loose bowel movements," so that "hooray . . . the more time you spend on the toilet, the better." On the subject of weight loss produced by bouts of diarrhea, she pontificates, "How else does fat leave your body? It doesn't magically absorb into the cosmos!" (In a sense, it does, in that body fat can be burned off as energy, or heat.)

Most of the academic research on dieting argues that not only are diets ineffective, but they can metabolically predispose the dieter to gain more weight than was lost. Dieting is only a temporary solution to weight gain. Studies have shown that the overwhelming majority of dieters regain the weight they lost within one year. Five-year follow-up studies indicate that only a small percentage of dieters are able to maintain their initial weight loss. The reason that weight loss is so difficult to maintain lies in the body's built-in adaptive mechanisms.

Our bodies are designed, through fat storage, to tolerate periods of starvation; our cave dwelling ancestors often went for weeks with little or no food. Those with plenty of stored fat in their bodies lived longer than those with smaller stores (survival of the fattest, you might say).

In our food-abundant nation, this storage mechanism is obsolete, but it exists nonetheless. Layers of fat that once insured survival are now the object of social intolerance and self-loathing. Ironically, the fat person of today would have been in an enviable position many years ago.

On a severely restricted diet (fewer than 1,200 calories per day) the metabolism decreases between 15 and 25 percent to make the body more fuel efficient. Fewer calories are then required to maintain a specific weight—a protective mechanism of the body designed to keep us from starving ourselves. Extreme dieting and fasting can thus paradoxically cause excessive deposits of fat.

Through a process called *hyperlipogenesis* (meaning unusually rapid conversion of foodstuffs to fats, or lipids), starvation and weight loss are often followed by an alteration of metabolism that, in turn, replenishes and even overloads fat stores. Numerous studies show that after repeated attempts at dieting, subjects burn fewer calories, are less active, and spend fewer calories on the same work than they'd spent before food restriction.

Hyperlipogenesis may be the cause of excessive hunger in dieters. Because the food is quickly removed from the bloodstream and stored as fat, the dieter feels unsatisfied until he has ingested sufficient quantities to maintain his blood sugar at a higher level. Therefore, the amount of food required to feel full far exceeds the body's actual requirements. Thus the individual either leaves the table hungry and frustrated, or eats until he feels comfortable, thereby foregoing his diet. This adaptive mechanism can be compared to drug tolerance in that greater amounts become necessary to produce the same effect; repeated periods of food restriction intensify the effect of hyperlipogenesis.

Many obese people actually become *more overweight* than if they had simply not dieted at all. This is because, during subsequent weight gains, metabolic stockpiles of fat that overcompensate for the original weight loss can result in the individual gaining more weight than was originally lost, even without overeating. Succinctly phrased by Dr. Gabe Mirkin, author of *Getting Thin—All About Fat*: (1983) "The best you can hope for from a diet is a temporarily thin body that's still shackled to a fat metabolism. Begin to eat normally, and the weight comes right back. Often with interest."

Most medical professionals agree that moderate, stable overweight is less threatening to an individual's health than repeated weight losses and gains. Studies indicate that cholesterol levels in the blood increase during periods of weight gain, and that fatty deposits are lodged inside the walls of coronary arteries. With subsequent weight gain, the blood vessels narrow even further. Thus the individual who continuously loses and regains weight is at *more risk for heart attack* than the individual who remains moderately overweight.

Body weight *stability* appears to be more significant for long-term health than other weight-related factors. Adults whose body weight has remained unchanged since the age of twenty-one (the time at which the musculoskeletal system is fully developed) have a reduced risk of obese-related diseases.

Harvard nutritionist Dr. Frederick J. Stare has studied the effects of weight loss and subsequent weight gain on the blood vessels of the heart. He states that damage to the blood vessels can occur with a regained weight loss of as little as ten pounds. Repeated cycles can lead to atherosclerosis, a progressive disease whereby arteries become silted up with fatty deposits. L. Louderback, author of *Fat Power: Whatever You Weigh Is Right*, offers worthwhile advice for us all: "If you are presently thin, do not get fat. If you are fat, try not to get fatter. But if you are not absolutely certain that you can sustain a lower weight for the rest of your life, do not attempt to lose weight."

If a fitness instructor demonstrates knowledge and understanding of how dieting can fail despite tremendous effort, his students will be greatly relieved. An affirmation that their size might not be entirely their fault will help them gain the self-confidence necessary to approach weight loss from a realistic perspective.

Brown Fat Theory

In the last few years new studies have suggested another possible explanation as to why some people will gain weight eating the same amounts of food that others will eat with no weight gain at all. Just as some people are predisposed to overweight due to a large number of fat cells (which contain a greater volume of lipids), it would also appear that some individuals are physiologically inclined to be lean due to large numbers of *brown fat cells*. These types of fat cells are full of blood vessels (which explains their dark color) and have a high metabolic activity potential. The blood vessels in these fat cells increase resting heat production. Unlike yellow fat, which is distributed throughout the body and can move about, brown fat is localized and cannot move. It is located between the shoulder blades, under the armpits, around the kidneys, and around the large veins and arteries near the heart. Brown fat functions as a blood warmer to protect the heart from becoming chilled (Mirkin, 1983).

Individuals with more brown fat cells are able to maintain their weight at optimum levels because the excess calories are burned off as heat (a process called *thermogenesis*). There is mounting evidence that fat people have fewer brown fat cells, and that the supply they have is less active than that of their lean peers. Individuals who have a small supply of inactive brown fat cells may store fat because there is no brown fat to waste it.

Further research is necessary before definite conclusions can be made about the relationship between brown fat cells and thinness or obesity. Yet in cases of individuals who are overweight despite normal eating habits, the role of brown fat cells appears to be significant.

The Relationship Between Inactivity and Fat, or, "Curse of the Couch Potato"

Inactivity is widely regarded as a serious problem for the obese. Sedentary lifestyles contribute greatly to weight gain, increased body fat, and lethargy. The Department of Health and Human Services report of June 1986 states that "obesity is primarily the result of low levels of physical activity rather than excess consumption of calories." Other studies have also concluded that overweight people do not eat more than persons of normal weight.

As a society we are immobilizing ourselves into a state of chubbyhood. The very gadgets invented to lighten our load are instead (physiologically speaking) weighing us down! Too often our free time is spent prostrate in front of the tube, a bowl of munchies strategically situated near its target zone. Less physical effort is nowadays required for survival, so more of our leisure time is devoted to avocations of casual observation (otherwise known as *vegetation*).

Many researchers point to inactivity as a major cause of obesity. Drs. Hans Kraus and Wilhelm Raab (cited in Kuntzleman & Consumer Guide Editors, 1978) have coined the term *hypokinetic diseases* to describe a number of diseases and disorders produced by insufficient motion. They contend that without activity, tension results, which can lead to emotional and physical dysfunction. Diseases resulting from stress include various metabolic maladies of which obesity is the most common. Other diseases aggravated by stress are gastrointestinal disorders, cardiovascular diseases, endocrine malfunctions, and musculoskeletal dysfunction. Thus it would appear that inactivity is a major link in the causative chain connecting obesity and disease.

When we are inactive, our bodies assume that there must be something wrong, so they "help" us by storing fat. This unfortunate assumption is probably another throwback to the times when frequent physical activity was necessary for survival. At one time in history if man was not continually on the move, you can bet something was amiss! Therefore, when we are idle for prolonged periods, our metabolisms will slow down to the point at which rolling out of bed is the best we can hope for (the old "use it or lose it" syndrome). Once we be-

gin to use our bodies as nature intended, our metabolisms and our muscles respond accordingly.

As I remind my classes time and again, our bodies are built for movement. Our many hundreds of muscles each have numerous functions besides movement, but it is movement that stimulates these functions. Muscles influence our circulatory, metabolic, and endocrine systems, our bones, and our posture. They serve as an emotional outlet for stress, thus creating the balance between our physical and emotional well-being. Spending great gobs of time resting on our laurels is not good for our physical well-being. The ability to move about freely is a privilege—one that should be taken advantage of, not taken for granted.

Health Risks

Research regarding obesity and disease is as diverse as it is controversial. While one study may argue that as little as 5 percent excess body fat is dangerous, another finds that an excess of as much as 40 percent doesn't always pose a threat to health. Some results are criticized because their methods are based on biased samples and confounded results. For example, certain studies conclude that fat people are physically and psychologically disabled. Critics point out that the researchers in these studies use only those subjects who are under stress, probably due to the social stigma attached to being fat. It is not reasonable to associate just one basic personality type as representing all obese people. If proper control groups are used with healthy, happy fat subjects who have favorable body images, research findings might be very different (Rodin, 1982).

A researcher's personal bias against fat often affects his methodology. The real risks involved in moderate overweight are not yet clear because scientific evidence often becomes clouded by prejudice. However, it is generally accepted throughout the medical and health professions that, above levels of 30 percent excess fat, there is a straight-line relationship between obesity and disease. The body just isn't equipped to handle vast overloads of fat for any length of time, and often breaks down under the strain.

Although being fat is not always the cause of degenerative illnesses, certain conditions related to fat are also related to many diseases. For instance, being fat may not of itself cause a heart attack, yet the existence of high levels of certain blood fats does contribute to heart attack. And fat people very often have high blood fat levels.

A personal observation might clarify this point: Most FFF students are moderately overweight and enjoy reasonably good health. They eat nutritious foods (occasional treats notwithstanding) and exercise regularly. But a few of them experience medical problems that stem from being seriously overweight.

One such student of mine is in her early thirties, and until recently had normal vitals, normal blood fat levels, and appeared to be in good health. Her biggest obstacle in maintaining good health is her extreme obesity. In class she is able to perform only a few of the exercises—it's hard to discern whether she simply tires easily or is uninspired to exercise (though she's been in the program over a year).

Results of her latest checkup indicate that this individual is a borderline Type II diabetic (a condition discussed later in this chapter). If she does not change her eating habits (which include binging and sugar addiction) she runs the risk of becoming critically ill. This woman appears to have tried everything to lose weight—from Overeaters Anonymous, to diet clinics, to exercise. Yet her weight hasn't altered by more than a few pounds—up or down—in over a year. Whatever her difficulty in losing the necessary weight to sustain a healthy life, her success has been negligible, and she risks serious, long-term health complications unless a complete and permanent dietary turnaround can be effected. If tenacity and willingness to try were the keys to weight loss, this lady could slip into a size ten.

The following topics relate to medical problems most frequently occurring in members of the FFF program. The instructor may find other health problems regularly appearing among her own participants, in which case he or she may wish to review specific material to become better informed in that area. A list of recommended reading material appears in the back of the book to assist you in your studies.

High Blood Pressure in FFF

The problem of high blood pressure is not unique to fat people. It affects one American in four. Our workdays are often hectic, while our leisure time is commonly spent immobilized. Busy schedules cause us to sacrifice nutrition for convenience foods, which can create havoc with our internal systems. The by-product of our new lifestyles is often a vascular system that plugs up with fat, making the smooth flow of blood and oxygen an uphill battle.

When I began screening the blood pressure of FFF members I was surprised to find out that more than 30 percent of them had high blood pressure (according to the American Heart Association, hypertension is 140/90). Many applicants were unaware of their condition. Some expressed disbelief because they'd had no symptoms (most people with HBP, in fact, have no physical symptoms).

When students require treatment to control HBP, it is of paramount importance that the instructor apprise the individual of the need to seek treatment. Follow-up questions should be asked periodically to insure that each participant is taking the medication as prescribed. I mention the latter point because a few of my students have complained that they'd gone off medication after experiencing adverse reactions. But physicians recommend that hypertensive patients *continue taking their high blood pressure medication until they've consulted with their doctor.* At that time it will be the physician's responsibility to make the necessary change in prescription or dosage.

High blood pressure (antihypertensive) medication can be lifesaving. It is not something that can be taken at the patient's convenience. In fulfilling your obligation as a fitness instructor, it would be unwise (and legally risky) to allow a hypertensive student who is not in control of her condition to enroll in your class. If she has been informed of the health risk and still decides not to seek treatment, neither the instructor nor the facility will wish to assume responsibility should any problems result from the exercises. (For more information on legal liability, see chapter 3.)

The good news is that it doesn't usually take much convincing for most of our students to seek medical advice. Once they have been told that their health is in jeopardy and that the physician's authorization before exercising is in their best interests, they will take appropriate measures. I have never lost a potential student because she didn't wish to be bothered with the protocol. I discuss how promising her future can be with proper treatment and regular exercise. But I also bring up the adverse possibilities of not assuming personal responsibility for one's health. We have only one chance at life. Once we've learned a few health tips that will enable us to sustain lengthier and more productive lives, it is unreasonable to assume that the end (good health) is not worth the means (a little self-discipline).

What is High Blood Pressure?

High blood pressure is a warning that the blood vessels are becoming silted with fatty deposits (atherosclerosis). As the arteries narrow, the heart must work harder to pump blood through the body. The greater the resistance (or the higher the fat content in the arteries), the higher the blood pressure.

This process can be compared to a garden hose that is partly covered at the tip. The water comes out of the uncovered half with greater force. Similarly, blood flowing through arteries that are partially blocked by fat or plaque must move under greater pressure. The increased pressure wears down the inner walls of the arteries, creating worn spots that are targets for the deposit of more fat or plaque. Eventually the arterial walls become so narrow that a blood clot (thrombus) might form. If the blood vessels in the heart become blocked, the result is a heart attack (coronary thrombosis or myocardial infarction). If the clot blocks the blood vessels in the brain, a stroke (cerebral thrombosis) results.

Approximately one-half of the deaths in the U.S. today are caused by heart attacks and strokes. Indeed, they are the leading causes of death (followed by cancer and then diabetes). For many obese individuals, extra calories end up as high cholesterol, which causes plaquing and high blood pressure.

Stress and Disease

Some people suffer no emotional trauma from being fat. For others, fat becomes the focus of all their problems. Such people frequently regard their body size as the only obstacle to their happiness: "My life would be perfect, if only I weren't fat." Sometimes fat is used consciously or subconsciously as a protective shelter against reality—it says to the world "I'm fat, therefore I needn't deal with anything more." Susie Orbach's *Fat Is a Feminist Issue* (1978) is an excellent treatise on the complex issue of obesity as a psychological tool.

Prejudice, discrimination, and social pressure to conform contribute to the psychological problems of the overweight (see "Societal Attitudes Toward Fat People" in this chapter). As you have seen, risk factors such as heart disease and gastro-

intestinal disorders are often stress related. Yet if the stigma of fat did not exist, the risk of stress-related illnesses associated with obesity might not be as great. I cite the following study as a case in point.

A study of an Italian-American, blue-collar community in Pennsylvania (Stout, Morrow, Brandt, & Wolf, 1964) showed both a high incidence of overweight and a very low incidence of death from heart attack. In this community obesity was socially acceptable. Its residents consumed a great deal of fat and wine and lived in a completely supportive environment. The study found, furthermore, that heart disease and diabetes levels in the community were below the average for slender Americans, all of which suggests that if all moral judgment about obesity were suspended, and overweight people were no longer pressured to conform to unrealistic models, they might actually be quite healthy.

Diabetes

Non-insulin-dependent, adult-onset diabetes (Type II) frequently occurs in obese men and women around the age of forty. It is caused by excess insulin produced by the pancreas. As mentioned in the section on "Pregnancy and Permanent Weight Gain," with the presence of excess insulin a large share of blood sugar is converted to fat and stored in fat cells rather than burned off as fuel. The breakdown of fats for fuel is inhibited by this process, and leads to a dependence on sugar as the major source of energy. The end result of this cycle is increased body fat.

It is estimated that 80 to 90 percent of adults having Type II diabetes are overweight. Fat people are vulnerable to this disease because of the resistance in their fat cells to the hormone insulin (see "Refined Carbohydrates," this chapter). Eventually their bodies become so insensitive to their ever-increasing supply of insulin that the insulin becomes ineffective in maintaining a balance of blood glucose levels.

Long-term damage from diabetes is caused by high blood sugar levels. Excess glucose can lead to capillary damage in the heart, kidney, retina, and nervous system. Excess glucose seems to make platelets (the blood's clotting mechanisms) stickier than they should be, leading to clotting of small blood vessels.

Although the reason is not yet completely clear, weight loss can often cure Type II diabetes.

The fatter the person, the fuller his fat cells, which makes them resistant to taking in more fat. The pancreas in such cases produces so much insulin that eventually it is ineffective for keeping either fat or sugar out of the blood. Losing weight empties some of the fat cells, allowing for a renewed response to insulin (Mirkin, 1983). Exercise also seems to increase sensitivity to insulin (this is discussed further in chapter 5, "Appetite Control"). As muscles strengthen they seek to increase their glycogen stores, requiring more sugar from the bloodstream. (See Figure 2.2 for a comparison of both blood sugar and insulin activity in normal weight and in obese individuals.)

Periodontal Disease

Because they eat more sugar, overweight individuals often have more dental problems than lean individuals. Refined sugar and white flour, from which all fiber is removed, build up easily on and between teeth. This concentration is conducive to bacterial fermentation and acid production, which weaken the structure of the teeth and gums.

Additional Health Risks

Other health risks attributed to excess body fat include damaged blood vessels, which can lead to heart attack and stroke; digestive disorders; respiratory ailments; enlarged heart; kidney problems; blood lipid disorders; malignant tumors of the ovaries and uterine lining in postmenopausal women; colon, rectal, and prostate cancer in men; and mechanical problems, particularly of the low back, hips, knees, and ankles (see FFF-FYI—Physical Limitations and Restrictions).

As the reader has seen, obesity is clearly a multifaceted problem with no easy solutions. Researchers are learning more and more about the complexities of overweight and its implications on health and well-being. It will be helpful for you, the instructor, to keep abreast of new findings in this field. Students will appreciate your knowledge and enthusiasm on their behalf.

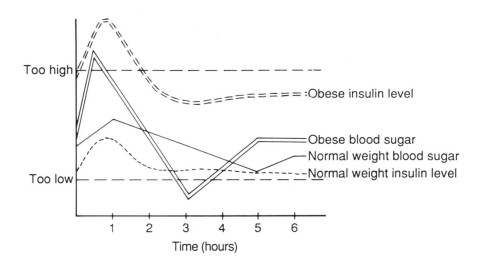

Figure 2.2   Effect of obesity on blood sugar and insulin. *Note.* **Adapted from *How to Lower Your Fat Thermostat* by D. Remington, G. Fisher, and E. Parent, 1983, Provo: Vitality House. Adapted with permission.**

Chapter

3

Broad Scope Program Development

The fitness industry is undergoing rapid change and increasing competition. In order to conduct a quality fitness program, today's fitness leader must be able to demonstrate much more than exercises. Nowadays serious fitness instructors attend numerous workshops to keep themselves informed about current research findings, nutritional information, and new trends in fitness. They must be acutely aware of legal responsibility and liability. The days of the homemaker conducting aerobics classes in her basement are over. Fitness has industrialized and professionalized into big business. To be successful you must be able to compete, and you can't compete without being informed and without understanding your market.

This chapter focuses on the many responsibilities of the successful fitness leader. The individual who chooses a career in fitness or in the health sciences must be multitalented and people oriented. If her career is to move forward, she will be expected to demonstrate (a) *versatility*—the ability to wear different hats, (b) *drive*—the ability to wear different hats at the same time, and (c) *determination*—the ability to wear different hats at

the same time and arrange them so cleverly that they make a fashion statement!

Initiating the Full Figure Fitness Program

For those readers who are affiliated with a YMCA, health management service wellness center, or fitness facility, convincing your director to offer the Full Figure Fitness program should not pose much of a problem. Whether the organization is for profit or not for profit, we all have budget demands that require some kind of income. It is the income potential that makes FFF so attractive to businesses.

Full Figure Fitness offers three things that are important to health promotion centers:

- *Community service.* The issue of overweight in the health and wellness field is usually addressed in terms of weight reduction and health risks. Few, if any, establishments offer a specific, healthful exercise plan for over-weight participants, in a completely accepting atmosphere. Facilities that do offer exercise classes usually bill them as "beginner fitness," and weight reduction is at least an implicit goal. Those who don't lose weight, or those who feel that they're beyond a "beginner's" stage, may have no other viable programming available to them.

Thirty-five percent of the population is overweight, and the rest of us know someone who is. These people are in need of activity, acceptance, and healthful lifestyle changes. But the advice they often receive is nebulous and negative: "Take better care of yourself—exercise and eat right!" The FFF plan affords the individual, as well as his physician, family, and friends, a specific, realistic plan of action instead of the vague "Do something!" approach.

- *Program enhancement.* By incorporating FFF into its program schedule, your facility will increase its fitness class enrollment (and profitability) significantly.

Remember, overweight men and women have tended to avoid exercise classes because of possible intimidation or discomfort. FFF precludes these possibilities by providing a program of sound exercise principles tailored to the specific needs of overweight people and a supportive, accepting atmosphere among others who share similar concerns.

- *Membership growth.* Initially, new participants may prefer to pay a nonmember rate rather than join a fitness facility. But as their self-confidence grows through the discipline of regular, hearty exercise, their desire also increases to participate in other activities offered by the facility. In our YMCA FFFers are often seen walking the track, swimming, or participating in water exercise classes. Such unabashed resolve usually begins with one student encouraging another to exercise: "I'll walk on the track if you'll join me." And a new member is born!

Independent instructors should contact community centers and explain the program in detail. I find that park and recreation commissions are very receptive to Full Figure Fitness, and those located in large cities are often willing to work with the instructor in locating a good facility in a well-populated area.

Health care professionals who would not instruct FFF, but who would like to refer patients or clients to the program, should contact nearby YMCAs, fitness centers, or health clubs to find out if there is an existing program. If not, simply suggest that they initiate one (if they are unfamiliar with FFF, show them a copy of this book!).

If you prefer an on-site program for your hospital, medical center, or the like, many facilities will provide you with a trained instructor to aid in its development and promotion. Introducing a new FFF program to your community is a challenge requiring salesmanship and professional know-how (you have to "know-how" your service is going to be received!). Once the director or officer of the establishment is convinced that the program will be profitable, and/or serve the needs of significant numbers of people, chances are that you can look forward to a long and rewarding experience with the Full Figure Fitness program.

Marketing the Full Figure Fitness Program

To offer a Full Figure Fitness program requires aggressive, creative marketing techniques. It is new, it is unique, and it is timely. Overweight adults represent a sizable market—more than 35 percent of the population—and one which is willing to spend a lot of money on physical improvements. Programs designed specifically for an overweight population are unusual. In fact, this market remains barely tapped by the fitness industry, in spite of the fact that the nation is beginning to strain its buttons!

FFF is in the right place at the right time. The media is highly receptive to new ideas, which makes marketing the program simpler. Below are a few of the features of FFF that make it attractive to journalists, reporters, and advertisers. With a little ingenuity, inexpensive publicity may be just a phone call away.

What Sets This Program Apart From the Others?

In their promotional material, conventional fitness programs often depict lean, good-looking young bodies as a sort of by-product of a healthy exercise plan. They suggest that leanness and beauty are both inherent to physical fitness. But this stereotype of the aerobic exerciser can create only a temporary interest in fitness for many. After all, the likelihood that regular workouts will make us look so terrific that we'll actually stop traffic is "slim" indeed! Most of us can expect to make only modest external adjustments. Without realistic goal setting and basic information on the genuine advantages of physical conditioning, participants can become disenchanted with exercise upon discovering that it does not always foster noticeable physical improvements.

The FFF Program Is Intelligent.   Our participants enjoy healthful, supervised exercise accompanied by fitness education. Students should receive weekly informative handouts about exercise, nutrition, stress reduction, and sportsmedicine to help keep them motivated to improve their conditioning.

The FFF Program Is Realistic.   It has a handle on the human condition, and doesn't give much credence to society's image of the beautiful people. Vive la différence! So there's no need for the program to promote the virtues of fitness beyond reality. Our market is real, live people with big bellies and bulging thighs. We don't promise to turn them into Ken and Barbie, or mold them into masters of their destiny. *Fitness feels better, it looks better, it helps us live longer.* And that is sufficient to satisfy people who "know better."

FFF is one of the few fitness programs that does not discriminate against fat people. We contend that *fat people can become more fit people without having to become thin people.* We use no intricate choreography that could produce awkwardness, discomfort, or embarrassment. There aren't any jumping or bouncing movements that could stress joints, tendons, and ligaments.

The FFF Program is Easy and Enjoyable.   For a few well-spent hours each week, participants work out in the company of their peers without intimidation or recrimination. The exercises are in a "follow-the-leader" style, so no one need concern themselves with anticipating steps. The exercise format is relaxed and easygoing.

When pursuing media coverage, emphasize each of these unique features in your program description. Be excited and compelling in your sales approach. Enthusiasm is catchy—so is the lack of it! It isn't always necessary to spend an enormous amount of money to capture the public's attention, but you have to possess something worth capturing! Media ears will perk up when they learn that you have something that can have

a favorable effect on more than 35 percent of their audience.

Target Markets

Announcements of FFF should cover areas within driving distance of the exercise facility (about ten miles in urban areas, fifteen miles in rural ones). My initial effort was through the "Tempo" section of our city newspaper. I telephoned the health columnist, Sue MacDonald, about the program and asked if she would be interested in mentioning it in her column. She was, and her article (reprinted below) generated over 100 phone inquiries. (Unfortunately, most of the people who called lived outside my area, and, at that time, there were no other FFF programs in the city. I learned to reach out only as far as my arms could stretch!) Many of the callers said that they found the program particularly appealing because they wanted and needed to get into an exercise program, but they didn't want to "exercise with skinny people"!

Overweight Workouts

Why is it that fitness classes seem to be filled to the brim with trim and skinny folks who look great in cutesy leotards?

Because many overweight people find the workouts too stressful on their already-stressed body frames, and because many are ashamed of their appearances.

The Clermont County YMCA, 2075 Frontwheel Dr., in Batavia, has started a fitness program for overweight people. It's called "Full Figure Fitness." The next sessions, one-hour coed workouts, begin Jan. 6. There will be morning and evening sessions.

Instructors have tailored a fitness program for persons who are overweight. Their emphasis is on exercise, not diets. Blood pressure screenings are conducted during workouts. Participants do physical activities that provide an aerobic workout without exerting tremendous pressure on joints, such as a 15-minute walk on the running track while doing arm exercises.

Soon after the article appeared, a local radio station called me requesting an interview. That interview aired several times, prompting more inquiries, and further improving business. Since then I have given several more interviews and enjoyed additional publicity for the program. Despite all this, because of other career commitments I have not been able to devote a great deal of time to promoting the program. Once the ball got rolling, it just sort of promoted itself. But you will find it necessary to dip into your advertising budget if more than a few months go by without the offer of free newspaper coverage—the public is quick to forget! Newspaper and radio coverage provide wide-range, no-cost publicity. In addition, articles and interviews provide a much more detailed description of the program than costly advertising.

Flyers and Brochures

Promotional flyers and brochures are another low-cost means of generating publicity. Because a variety of fitness programs are offered in my city, I wanted my FFF flyers to stand apart. For high visibility, we photographed an attractive, overweight woman wearing workout clothes. The photo covered the entire length of the page. (A sample flyer and brochure, with space for the name, address, and phone number of your facility are included in Appendix A.)

FFF literature can reach a vast number of people when distributed properly. There are many services that cater to overweight patients and clientele. In addition, many stores and shops are patronized by overweight people who might be interested in reading about the program. I have listed several businesses that could be helpful in promoting FFF. But before making personal visits to drop off flyers, first call and request permission from the store manager; some establishments may have policies precluding such distribution.

Whenever possible, I recommend meeting personally with the directors of professional services to explain the program. Through appointments or phone conversations I've been able to explain FFF to many professionals, who often express their enthusiasm and their willingness to refer clients and patients. Since first impressions are important in making connections, be prepared to articulate your program succinctly and proficiently before dialing. Jot down a few of the major points you wish to convey. Try to schedule an appointment. If that isn't possible, state your message briefly and directly, and thank your contact for his or her time.

The following shops and services are excellent sources of potential advertising for the program:

Hospital lobbies
Nutrition services
Sportsmedicine clinics
Health promotion services of hospitals
OB-GYN offices
Medical facilities
Clothing shops for large sizes
Weight loss centers
Chiropractic clinics
Eating disorder clinics
Community bulletin boards

Quid Pro Quo—(You Scratch My Back) . . . When you ask someone for promotional assistance, be prepared to offer something in return. For example, in exchange for carrying your promotional material and/or referring their own patients or customers to your business, offer them an opportunity to display *their* literature on your program site or to refer *your* students to their place of business.

Display Advertising

Display advertising is expensive, but it can attract many people to the program. It is more expedient to run a large display ad in your local paper than to run a smaller (comparably priced) ad in your metropolitan newspaper. Promotions that blanket areas well outside reasonable traveling distance can be a waste of money. Advertising in the metropolitan newspaper is worth the expense only if your FFF program will run in several different locations throughout that city.

Marketing to Men

Due to the sensitive nature of FFF, at least one all-female class is recommended. But don't be discouraged from developing either an all-male program or a coed FFF. There are plenty of men who feel similarly ostracized from society or assume they're too fat to participate in an exercise class. A feasibility study to determine the market for an all-male or a coed program would help you arrive at a clearer picture of whether or not such a program might be successful. If you are employed by a fitness facility, post a sign-up sheet for overweight men interested in a special exercise class. If you are not, advertise the program to both overweight men and women.

If you determine that an all-male class is warranted, you might be advised to change the name of the program to "Big Men's Workout" or something that conveys a macho image. (I know it's the eighties, but trust me—men won't go for the name ''Full Figure Fitness'' in an all-male class!) A flyer for a men's program also appears in Appendix A.

I think it is important to leave open the possibility of men in the program. I don't know of any other exercise programs for overweights that include men. (It wasn't long ago that all aerobics classes were made up of women only. That has changed, and now men and women enjoy aerobic exercise together.) An all-male or coed FFF program is a unique idea. It may take time before the idea catches on, just as with aerobic workouts, but I believe a continuous effort to promote the program to men is worthwhile.

Meticulous Marketing

Each step of the FFF program must be carefully considered and well-executed. Hastily drawn plans often suffer discouraging ends. Draft an outline of your plan of action and make adjustments as necessary before implementing your ideas. The more organized the program from start to finish, the more likely it will be successful.

As you have seen, the target audience for FFF is very accessible. The program will appeal to many overweight individuals who will be grateful for the opportunity to exercise in comfortable surroundings. FFF will also appeal to a number of health care professionals who will be pleased to refer their patients and clients to a program that affords them dignity and respect.

Legal Liability

As if planning, organizing, developing, training, marketing, and motivating were not enough, today's fitness leaders must also learn the legal ramifications of exercise instruction. But once again, organization and forethought can help minimize negative possibilities.

Before teaching any fitness program, be certain that you have liability coverage. Most fitness facilities will include you under their insurance umbrella, but rather than make assumptions, find out for sure. If you are an independent instructor, talk to your insurance agent about an insurance rider on your personal policy. If you belong to a professional organization such as Aerobic Fitness Association of America (AFAA) or International

Dance Idea Association (IDEA), liability insurance might be available to you.

In Appendix B there are a few simple forms to use, and some steps to follow, to protect yourself from the possibility of a lawsuit:

1. *Health History Form* (see page 63). Advise participants of the importance of their honesty in completing this form. If they fail to report an existing condition, they may be endangering their health.
2. *Application and Medical Clearance Form* (see page 64). The top half of this form includes the student's statement of interest in participating in an exercise program and the instructor's request for medical clearance. The bottom half, to be filled out by the physician, states either approval, disapproval, or exercise restrictions.
3. *Waiver, Release, and Indemnity Agreement* (see page 62). This document informs the participant of potential risks inherent to the fitness program. In the event of injury or death, the instructor and facility are exempted from liability. Waivers and informed consent forms aren't legally enforceable, but may deter the individual from filing a claim in the event of an injury.
4. *Careful Exercise Instruction, Demonstration, and Observation*. The leader has an obligation to her students. They know little about proper exercise, and trust that she knows more. Instructors can't just pop into a brand-new exercise program, turn on the music, and begin the workout assuming that nothing will go wrong. Don't assume anything—play it safe by thinking through all the possibilities.

In order to reduce your chances of being sued, explain proper exercise form and technique, target heart rates, and so on. Demonstrate the exercises before asking your students to do them; monitor their performance and make adjustments where necessary. Avoid exercises if you are unsure of their safety or efficacy. (I have a little saying for exercise uncertainties: ''When in doubt, don't!'') Pay close attention to exercise dos and don'ts presented in chapter 4.

What Determines Negligence?

Most lawsuits against fitness leaders involve negligence. When determining whether or not an individual was negligent, the judge and jury must assess:

1. *Presence of duty.* Instructors have legal obligations to their students. According to the *Coaches Guide to Sport Law* (Nygaard & Boone, 1985) the judicial system states that we have a duty to provide our participants several safeguards. They are:
   - Adequate supervision.
   - Sound planning.
   - Proper warning of inherent risks in the activities and dangers of improper techniques.
   - Safe environment. Be sure that the workout area is clean, dry, and free of obstacles.
   - Participant evaluation to determine any limitations.
   - First aid. Establish emergency medical procedures.
2. *Breach of duty.* Did the instructor fail to do what he should have?
3. *Cause of injury.* Did the instructor's own failure cause the injury?
4. *Extent of injury.* How much damage was done?

Each of the four factors listed above must be present before an instructor can be proven to have been negligent. But it is certainly more practical to avoid a nasty court battle through prudent planning than to risk paying the price later for your carelessness.

'Move' Music

FFF appeals to a wide range of ages and musical tastes. Although the movements are not choreographed, good background music is essential for pacing and for charging up energy.

When choosing music, you may find it's fun to include hits that span several generations and that represent diverse musical styles. Music from today's Top 40 is fine, but you can find toe-tapping tunes anywhere—don't limit yourself only to contemporary rock and roll! If you need assistance in selecting music, ask an experienced aerobic dance instructor, or check with your local record store manager.

The tempo during the aerobic phase should be a little faster than moderate—about 130 to 150 beats per minute (if you are unfamiliar with counting bpms, talk to an aerobics instructor). Try to keep the rhythm of each selection the same. Practice exercising to each song before leading the class to insure an easy-flowing, continuous pace. Remember, if the movements seem fast to you, they'll seem a lot faster to someone much bigger, particularly if that person must sustain a rapid-fire pace for the full twenty minutes. Floor work tempo is slower—about 120 bpm.

Warm-up music should be cheerful and energizing, but not too fast. "Hooked on Classics" or "Hooked on Swing" music is effective in getting exercisers into the right workout mood. I play two warm-up pieces: the first for stationary warm-ups, the second for stretches at the wall. Soft, easy cool-down music is truly appreciated by FFFers. The cool-down signals the close of another hardworking hour. It's time to relax and let go, so it's important that the music convey that message.

Classical music can be very soothing during the cool-down, but my personal preference is soft jazz. Jazz artists have a knack for creating music to get lazy by. My favorite cool-down piece is Grover Washington's "In the Name of Love" (on the album *Winelight*). Most students emit sighs of relaxed relief upon hearing its soft, gentle tones.

Putting together an hour of diverse music every couple of months isn't easy. But it can really pay off to keep your people funking to the new tunes and beebopping down memory lane!

Obtaining Music Rights

Exasperating though it may be, an instructor cannot legally turn on the tape he or she has spent hours recording and commence the exercise class without proper authorization. U.S. copyright laws protect songwriters, players, and publishers. Two organizations have the authority to license the rights to the music you play. The American Society of Composers, Authors, & Publishers (ASCAP), and Broadcast Music, Inc. (BMI) each provide a single license to use all of the song titles in their respective libraries. Because an artist may switch from one organization to the other, it is advisable to purchase a license from each.

The annual license fee for ASCAP for seventy-five students or less is $46.17. BMI's annual fee for 1,500 square feet or less is $60.00. Therefore, an annual fee of $106.17 will cover all of your facility's responsibilities, and may save someone between

$250 and $50,000 *per song* if you are caught infringing a copyright. The facility owner, not the instructor, is responsible for the music played in his or her establishment and must have the license. If you lease or rent space, the building owner is responsible, although both of you may be named in a lawsuit.

Proper licensing buys the right of the instructor to compile numerous songs on one tape as long as that tape is not sold. For additional information on music licensing, cail ASCAP in New York (212-595-3050) or Los Angeles (213-466-8401). BMI has a toll free number (800-523-0237, or in California 800-642-4422).

Commonly Asked Questions by Full Figure Fitness Participants

Throughout the program, students will ask many questions about all sorts of health-related issues. The following are those which I hear asked most often. More questions will undoubtedly arise and with some it will be necessary to seek the advice of an expert.

Question: My doctor prescribed a diuretic to get rid of the excess water in my system. Am I exempt from your suggestion to drink eight to ten glasses of water each day, since I have too much already?

Answer: Absolutely not. Diuretics work in combination with water. When our systems lack a sufficient supply, water is stored in the tissues rather than passed through, creating puffiness and swelling. People who store water need to drink more of it so that it won't be hoarded by the tissues.

Question: I have arthritis. Is this program okay for me?

Answer: First check with your doctor. Most physicians encourage arthritic patients to exercise so that their joints don't deteriorate further from lack of use. Range of motion exercise keeps muscles viable and joints lubricated, which enhances movement. If land exercise is too painful, try exercising in the water.

Question: Are strength training machines good for fat people?

Answer: Nautilus equipment is excellent to stretch and strengthen muscles. But before beginning a weight training regimen, the obese exercise beginner should concentrate first on cardiovascular conditioning and endurance training. Overweight people generally have sufficient strength in their large muscles (those in the arms and legs) to support their size. But their aerobic capacity and muscular endurance are usually diminished by inactivity. Increasing the ability of the cardio-respiratory system to utilize oxygen and burn fat for fuel should take precedence over strength training.

Furthermore, without restricting food intake, body weight will likely increase during the first weeks of weight training as heavy muscle tissue develops. The fact that the weight represents muscle, not fat, is of little comfort to someone who lives by the scale and hopes to reduce body weight through exercise. Strength training doesn't alter the metabolism as significantly as aerobic training, so unless a person reduces his intake, the size of his muscles may increase without a dramatic decrease in body fat. The result can be clothes that actually fit tighter after training than before.

Question: I've been exercising for months and haven't lost a pound. Should I exercise more?

Answer: If people retain poor nutritional habits, they may still consume more calories than their exercise burns off. Furthermore, some bodies are reluctant to give up fat, perhaps having adjusted to a very slow metabolism that doesn't use much energy.

Another reason for not losing weight through exercise could be that the individual isn't exercising aerobically. Overweight bodies adjust to the rigors of exercise like anyone else's, only not as quickly. As their bodies adapt, the intensity of the workout needs to be increased. When pulse rate has decreased from its previous exercise rate, it's time to put more into your workout, or to work out more.

If weight loss is your goal, moderating the intake of nutritious foods in conjunction with some form of daily exercise might be necessary. But don't lose sight of the many other benefits of exercise. Physical and mental well-being are also important components of a healthy body.

Question: After taking FFF should I be ready for something more difficult?

Answer: FFF is designed to improve all the components of fitness on an ongoing basis—"graduating" to a more intense exercise program is not necessary. The combination of low-impact aerobics and continuous arm movement allows the student to advance at her own pace. In the early stages of training, she may need to sit one out occasionally. As her fitness level increases, she can use wrist weights or increase the intensity of her workout through continuous, controlled arm and leg movements. Low-impact aerobics provides a cardiovascular workout through the use of large muscle groups—weight is lifted by tightly controlled muscles rather than thrust off the floor to a forceable landing. FFF is low impact—not low level!

Question: I've read that too much water is harmful, yet we are urged to consume mass quantities. Can we be getting too much?

Answer: It's extremely doubtful. The notion that too much water is harmful evolved from problems of endurance athletes who were consuming eight to twelve gallons in a twenty-four-hour period and experiencing certain physiological imbalances. Few people can tolerate that much fluid, so it really doesn't become an issue in the FFF program.

Muscles are 70 to 75 percent water. Exercise builds muscle. Therefore, if we are going to exercise, we need more water. In addition, exercise produces body heat, which makes us sweat, further warranting the consumption of water. (Special note—beverages such as cola, coffee, juice, and so on are *not* adequate replacements for water!)

Because fat contains very little water (about 25%), overweight individuals have less water in their bodies than individuals of normal weight. (Overweight adults average 45 percent body water and normal weight adults 50 to 55 percent.) Lack of sufficient body fluids can produce an array of maladies. So drink up! As a reminder to drink water, I give my new students a small piece of carboard separated into a 'Yes' side and a 'No' side. On the 'No' side I attach 8 paper clips, their instructions are to replace a 'No' side clip to the 'Yes' side with each glass of water consumed. By the end of the day, the 'NO' side should be empty.

Chapter

4
The Full Figure Fitness
Exercise Program

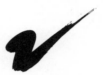

Before the first workout you will need to go over a few key points with your participants. You need to be sure that everyone gets the safest possible workout, and you can do this by providing some guidelines for self-monitoring. In Appendix C you will find a "Welcome to Full Figure Fitness" handout that can be distributed the first day of class. Of course, this should be retyped onto your business stationery. This handout gives some general advice for monitoring one's own workout. I advise new students to begin a 'fitness file' to retain distributional material from class as well as desired magazine or newspaper items on fitness and health. You will also need to teach participants to calculate and monitor their own exercise heart rates. The steps outlined in Appendix D will help you do that.

The Class Format

So that students can obtain significant results from training, the FFF program should be offered three times weekly. If classes are held less often, students must scramble for another activity that will provide the same benefits or else remain "stuck" at a maintenance level. Overweight exercisers are very attentive devotees of the FFF program, but they won't often seek additional unstructured exercise opportunities.

The format followed in the FFF program consists of the warm-up, cardiorespiratory or aerobic phase, water break, brief stretching, floor exercises, and cool-down. Experience has taught that the aerobic phase should come before floor work. There are several reasons for this: Overweights have to move a lot of body mass during the workout, and floor exercises can produce such achiness in some that they must really struggle to do anything more. Aerobic activity in the latter portion of the program then becomes arduous and unpleasant. It is more practical to "aerobicize" during the first half of class when participants' energy levels are highest. Furthermore, when aerobics follow the warm-up, muscles are well heated and so more receptive to the demands placed on them during the later strength and endurance training. And finally, with this format students do not need to keep changing positions from supine to standing, as both muscular strengthening and cool-down exercises are performed primarily from a recumbent position.

Exercises should be challenging—*avoid the temptation to underexercise fat people.* With proper instruction before class, each participant will pace him or herself appropriately. Keep a few chairs around the room for those who will need to rest.

Be certain that both form and purpose of each strengthening and stretching exercise are explained thoroughly. Most of your participants will have little understanding of what the exercises are supposed to achieve. You should take the time to explain

- Why proper form is necessary,
- What muscles are being worked, and
- Where a particular exercise or stretch should be felt.

You must never assume your participants understand the relevance of your demonstrations.

Warm-Up Exercises

A good warm-up takes 5 to 10 minutes. Begin warming up with deep-breathing exercises. Inhale as the arms rise outward and upward, exhale as the arms come down. Follow with light stretches such as those suggested below. Advise students to hold the stretching muscle in control. Jerking or bouncing against a joint is contraindicated, but old-fashioned methods might still be ingrained in some, so watch each student carefully.

A list of recommended warm-up exercises follows. The instructor should improvise modifications to these routines whenever she feels confident that such modifications are safe and effective.

Neck and Shoulders

Semicircles: With chin, beginning with head down. Roll head to the right, down, left, down (never roll the head backward).

Head Turns: Slowly roll the head toward the left shoulder, then toward the right shoulder.

Shoulder Rolls: Roll shoulders forward a few times, then reverse. Move shoulders together up and down; move alternate shoulders up and down. Squeeze shoulders together to the front and then to the back.

Arms: Repeat Each Movement Several Times

Arm Press: Extend arms to the sides, parallel to floor, palms facing behind you, gently pressing arms back.

Arm Circles: Rotate arms forward a few times, then reverse. (The circles should not be too wide—keep the movement controlled.)

Arm Press Side to Side: Cross left arm over toward right, palm up, and press out; alternate arms.

Overhead Reach: Alternating arms, reach toward the ceiling.

Elbows In, Arms Out: With hands at chest and elbows out, press shoulders back, followed by arms extended (parallel to floor).

Torso

Gentle Twist: As shown in Figure 4.1, clasp fingers, raise arms overhead. Gently twist to the right, hold (about six seconds), then slowly twist left and hold. Clasp fingers, arms down, plié (place feet and legs apart, knees bent), then bring arms up while straightening. Repeat four times. Advise class to keep their feet and knees aligned, or pointing in the same direction—if knees are bent outward, feet should point out; if knees are straight ahead, feet should be straight ahead.

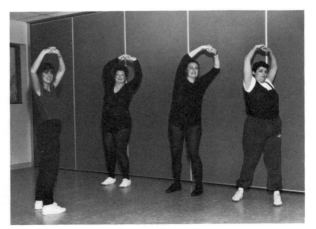

Figure 4.1   Gentle twist

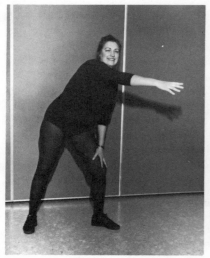

Figure 4.2   Stretch forward

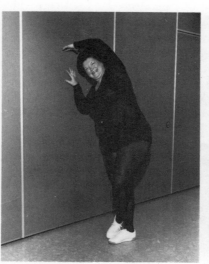

Figure 4.3   Side stretch

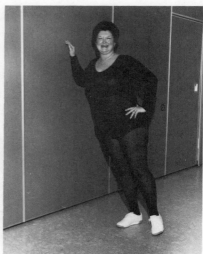

Figure 4.4   Hip stretch

Stretch to the Side With Arm Overhead.   Keep hand on thigh to help push back up to starting position (takes pressure off lower back).

Stretch Forward.   Bend knees slightly, reach out to opposite side, opposite hand resting on thigh, push off from thigh, to straight reverse (see Figure 4.2).

Wall Stretch Series

Stretches at the wall are especially appropriate for FFF students. The wall provides support, which facilitates warm-ups for the lower body. Students avoid the awkwardness of attempting to balance their weight. Be sure to monitor your students' body alignment, particularly at the feet and knees.

Side Stretch: Place arm overhead with outside ankle crossed over inside ankle with both feet flat on the floor (see Figure 4.3) to enhance the stretch.

Hip Stretch (see Figure 4.4):   Rest forearm against wall, legs together. Slowly lean hip toward wall as far as it will stretch comfortably. When properly executed, the hips will not be in alignment with the rest of the body. Stretch should be felt from the ilium (tensor fasciae latae muscle) to the tibia. This area is called the iliotibial tract (see Figure 4.5), which helps stabilize the knee joint. The hip stretch is especially important in FFF because it helps prevent *iliotibial band syndrome* (see Figure 4.5), or

snapping of the knee, which occurs frequently in overweight individuals.

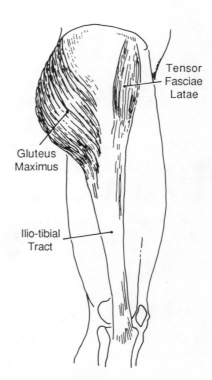

Figure 4.5   The iliotibial band

Calf Stretch (see Figure 4.6):   Face wall, press forearms against it with elbows at shoulder level. Move one foot up to wall, bending knee. Rear foot and leg should be facing straight ahead, with knee nearly locked. Both feet are flat on floor. After about 10 seconds, bend the back knee slightly to stretch the soleus muscle along the Achilles tendon. Switch legs.

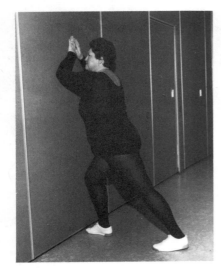

Figure 4.6   Calf stretch

Pectoral Stretch/Back Stretch (see Figure 4.7): This is similar to the cat stretch, which is performed on the hands and knees. Begin by standing an arm's length away from the wall, hands at chest level. Bend forward keeping hips tucked in, abdominal muscles tight (this will stretch the lower back). After several seconds, let the back sink in, releasing abdominal contraction, and pressing the hips

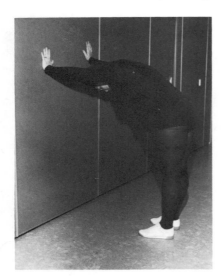

Figure 4.7   Pectoral stretch

out (this will stretch the pectoral muscles, hamstrings, and calf muscles). Hold briefly. "Walk" hands up the wall to an erect position. Extension and flexion exercises are especially important in stretching and strengthening muscles of the lower back and abdomen. Extension exercises are often omitted in classes, which can cause lower back muscles to become overstretched and weak.

Quadricep Stretch (see Figure 4.8):   Maintain balance by leaning shoulder against the wall (although students should challenge their balancing abilities occasionally by attempting this exercise with no support). Raise heel toward buttock, grasp ankle (very obese students may need to grab onto the back of their shoe or sock if they cannot reach their ankle). Bring heel close to buttock while pressing leg back (to stretch hip flexor). Reverse.

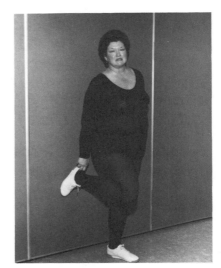

Figure 4.8   Quadriceps stretch

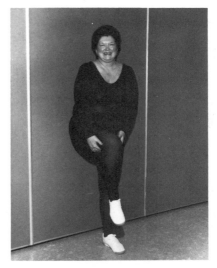

Figure 4.9   Shin and ankle warm-up

Shin and Ankle Warm-Up (see Figure 4.9): Lean back against wall. Raise bent leg slightly, grasp sides of thigh. Circle toes several times in each direction. Then alternately point and flex the feet. For strengthening the ankles, turn foot in, then out (inversion and eversion); repeat several times. Be sure to demonstrate this as it appears in the figure. Avoid pulling your knee to your chest, since this may not be possible for some participants.

Cardiorespiratory Phase (Aerobics)

The aerobic workout should last for 20 minutes. Since the FFF program is ongoing, with the exception of the first session (8–10 weeks) both beginners and advanced students will share the same program. The first two weeks of the first session should be limited to 12-15 minutes of low-impact aerobics. By the third week, the aerobic section should be 20 minutes long. Keep in mind, however, that only the first 8-week session will progress in the duration of the cardiorespiratory segment. In subsequent sessions the aerobic component should last the full 20 minutes. Most of your students will soon become "regulars," who have obtained a significant training effect from their aerobics. It would be unfair to revert to a low-level class every new session just to accommodate the new people. Exercises should be demonstrated primarily to the level of the majority. Intelligent instruction on "how to" and "how not to" will assist the new students in adjusting to their capabilities and limitations.

Try to schedule time before each new session to explain the program, and to demonstrate step calls to the new students. Advise new members to rest when they are tired (remember to keep chairs handy about the room), and to take a break as necessary (train, don't strain). Never allow students to work so hard that they must pant or gasp for air. Try to keep the new members closest to you during the first couple of weeks so that you can monitor form and breathing, and be available if they require assistance.

Free-Form, Low-Impact, High-Intensity Workouts

Low-impact aerobics (one foot on the floor at all times) emphasizes both safety and spirited energy. The recent discoveries of physiology and sports-medicine regarding injury from high-impact aer-

obics are making low-impact converts out of many participants *and* instructors. Low-impact aerobic workouts can accommodate all levels of fitness safely and effectively, which makes them an excellent exercise medium for an overweight population.

Exercisers are in better control and more apt to work at their own levels in a freestyle, low-impact regimen. Rather than bounding off the floor and landing with a force greater then three times body weight, students obtain a training effect through the shifting of their body weight and the use of large muscle masses in the legs and arms. Continuous arm movements are much more significant to maintaining target heart rates in this form of exercise. Aerobic experts believe that another significant advantage to low impact is that students are more often able to sustain the target heart rate for the full twenty to thirty minutes.

Low-impact aerobics has a tremendous number of variations that incorporate different arm movements with different steps. As coordination improves, students have a great time trying new routines. When a student who's had difficulty coordinating a particular movement finally masters it, she often sings out "I got it!" and enjoys a rousing cheer from her classmates.

However, no exercise is without risks. Body alignment, muscle control, and fluidity of motion are extremely important in low-impact aerobics (see "Special Considerations" in chapter 5). Quick, jerky movements, sudden turns, or pivots place tremendous pressure on tendons, joints, and ligaments, particularly of the hips and legs. This is especially significant for overweights, whose hips and legs must support unevenly distributed, excessive body weight. A greater emphasis must be placed on body awareness and coordination.

Exercise movements should be simple, energetic, and versatile. Encourage lots of hand clapping and hearty whoops to keep enthusiasm high and students constantly on the move. Change the movements frequently so that the class is always alert. (Sometimes I'll start chatting during the exercises and forget to change steps. Invariably someone will call out, "Hey, Bonnie, your needle is stuck!" Restraint is not one of our strong suits.)

Proper demonstration is crucial, as the class will follow the instructor's lead regardless of its appropriateness. If she tends to bounce and swing, the class will too, even if she has urged them not to. Unlike choreographed movements, which require concentration, free-form exercise necessitates only "copycatting" the movements of the instructor. Consequently, members of freestyle classes often turn off their thinking and move exactly as they see their leader moving. (If you've ever raised your hand to scratch your nose while leading exercises, and watched as a sea of hands curved upward, you know what I mean!)

Rate of progression will depend upon the individual. Initially your students should not be expected to keep their arms elevated for more than a few repetitions of a movement. As they tire, they will rest their arms at their sides or use smaller, less concentrated movements in their exercises. By the time they begin exercising, if properly guided, each will know when to slow down. As students progress, they should be encouraged to keep moving, and to make their movements bigger and more forceful. One-pound wrist weights are recommended for those in want of a more physically challenging workout.

Aerobic Movements

Posture should remain erect, and abdominal muscles should be tight throughout the aerobic section—students will need frequent reminders to ''pull it in!''

Step Kick (see Figure 4.10):   Alternating legs, kick out in time to the music. Opposite arm reaches out in front.

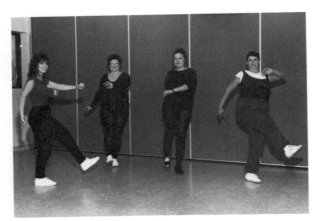

Figure 4.10   Step kick

Knee Lift, Arms Up (see Figure 4.11):   The knee lift has many variations. Arms can reach up, pull down, alternate up and down, and so on.

Overhead Pull (see Figure 4.12):   Arms overhead, pull apart as you step to one side (toes up), bring arms together as you step to the other side. Another variation begins with arms alternating up and down with each step.

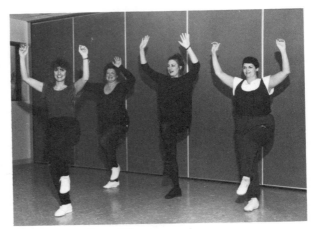

Figure 4.11   Knee lift, arms-up

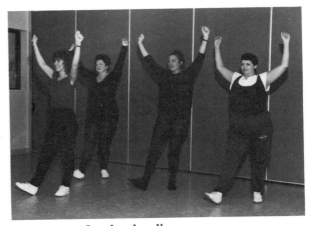

Figure 4.12   Overhead pull

Hopscotch (see Figure 4.13):   Arms out at sides, raise heel in back toward opposite hand, reverse. The hopscotch can also be done with a foot out in front, but this may be difficult for extremely overweight participants.

Grapevine (see Figure 4.14):   Step behind, step, kick, reverse direction.

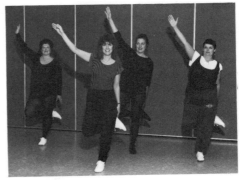

Figure 4.13   Hopscotch

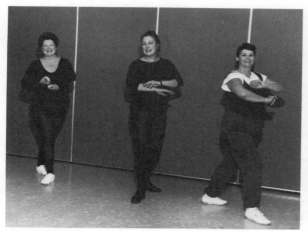

Figure 4.14   Grapevine

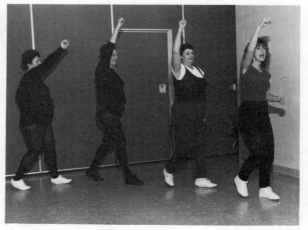

Figure 4.16   Circle walking

Circle Walking

Circle walking (walking single file in a circle around the floor) is an excellent low-impact adjunct. It can be incorporated into the daily exercise routine, or it can be used sporadically as an exercise variation. As in low-impact aerobics, arm movements are important in circle walking to help keep participants' heart rates at target levels. Some variations of arm movements include the following: overhead punches (see Figures 4.15 and 4.16); forward punches; airplane arms; pumping arms up and down; arm circles; triceps press (bend elbows, then extend arms back; repeat); and hands pressed together behind back.

There are many variations for the legs as well, including these: marching steps; ponies; step-kicks; steps into and out of the circle (step in, two, three, clap, and back, two, three, clap); steps and a hop (step, two, three, hop); four steps left and then right while facing inside the circle; grapevine left and right in circle formation; and so on. After several minutes of moving in the same direction, turn around and circle walk the other way.

Instructors should familiarize themselves with the wide variety of possible movements in low-impact aerobics by observing several different classes in person and/or on video. Many articles have been written about the relatively new concept of low-impact aerobics. I encourage instructors to read the literature and to practice the exercise steps themselves to music so that they have a clear understanding and mastery of this most important section of the program.

It often takes a few tries before everyone is moving together, but when we are, we can give the Solid Gold Dancers and the Rockettes a run for their money! And when we can't seem to pull it together, we can always poke fun at ourselves for having a bunch of rubber legs!

Pulse Check

After the cardiorespiratory workout, students should keep moving as they check their pulse rates (sudden stops can produce dizziness and nausea as blood pools in the lower extremities). A few students will be unable to locate their pulse and will require assistance. Pulses will be noticeably stronger after several weeks of regular physical activity.

Break

In an hour-long program, students should be allowed a brief water break (2-3 minutes) at the half-

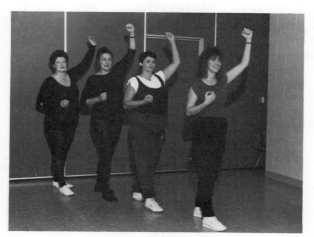

Figure 4.15   Circle walking

hour mark. Students will be hot, sweaty, and tired following aerobics, and this short break will be very refreshing. Urge them to drink slightly more water than they need to quench their thirst (many overweight adults do not consume enough water, but incorrectly assume that they are getting sufficient liquids through coffee, colas, and the like).

Ask your students to remain standing during the break. Immediately after exercise, the body begins to cool down. If they sit down, there's a chance they might become dizzy or light-headed when they stand. For this reason, it is also inadvisable to steam, sauna, or shower immediately after a vigorous workout. Give the body time to cool down completely.

Floor Work

In the first couple of weeks, before sitting down after the workout, take another pulse check. Students should be at or below 17 beats using a ten-second count (about 100 bpm). Postaerobics is an excellent time to lead the class through some luxurious slow stretches to soothe and relax their tense muscles. Stretching and relaxing should be partners for life, so teach the students to *allow*, rather than force, a long, easy stretch. Perform seated stretches for about 4 minutes, or the length of one song.

Back and Hip Stretch (see Figure 4.17): In a cross-legged position, reach across body (note the varying levels of flexibility); cross legs the other way and reach opposite arm across. This exercise stretches the back and hips.

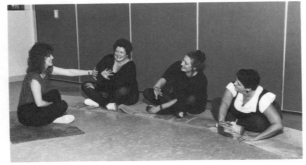

Figure 4.17 Back and hip stretch

Inner Thigh Stretch (see Figure 4.18): Bend knees, place feet in front of you, soles together. Gently press knees toward floor.

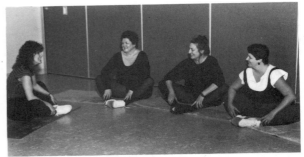

Figure 4.18 Inner thigh stretch

Sit and Reach (see Figure 4.19): Bend one leg (knee outward on the floor) and reach out toward extended leg; reverse. Be sure foot is flexed, toes pointed up for proper hip and knee alignment. This exercise stretches the calf, hamstring, and buttock muscles. (Note: It is unnecessary, and often unwise, to lock the knee joint when stretching. The knee joint ligaments can become overstretched and susceptible to injury.) Other seated stretches include the following: straddle position (legs out) with side stretch (ear toward knee), side reach (nose toward knee), or forward reach (feet flexed as arms reach out); side stretch with both arms overhead; overhead reach with arms clasped overhead, torso slowly twisting to the left, hold, and then to the right. *When executing a forward reach (seated or standing), students should push off from their thigh to straighten. This reduces strain on the lower back.*

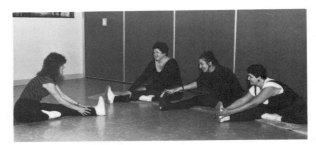

Figure 4.19 Sit and reach

Repetitions, Sets, and Progression

At first, students will be able to complete one set of eight repetitions before needing a rest. After three weeks, advance to two sets of eight repetitions per exercise set before each brief rest. Individuals will vary greatly in their adaptation to exercise (some may never adjust!), but most will demonstrate sufficient improvement within three weeks to warrant more challenging exercises and added reps.

Abdominal Strengthening

At least 5 minutes should be spent doing floor work. Begin the floor work with abdominal exercises, as these are the most difficult for overweight individuals and it is best to do them after a few minutes of stretching.

Abdominal exercises are of particular importance to overweight individuals, as they very often have poor muscle tone in this area. Abdominal strength reduces the low back pain suffered by many of our students.

Curl Up for Rectus Abdominis Muscles: With knees bent, feet flat on floor, and fingers gently supporting back of head, curl up slightly, and then lie back only as far as the scapula (middle of shoulders). Avoid bringing the head down to the floor, as neck pain will render the exercise extremely difficult to repeat. To alleviate neck discomfort (which is most severe during the first few weeks of conditioning), after each abdominal series, have the students lie back and roll their heads from side to side.

Working slowly, with tightly contracted abdominals and buttocks throughout, is the key to abdominal strengthening in overweight people. If you are exercising to a tempo, curl up and down

to alternate beats to keep the motion slow and concentrated.

Variations (see Figures 4.20a and b) include raising and lowering the torso while grasping the sides of the raised leg, or using a chair to support the legs while performing a series of abdominal curls. Another interesting variation is to drape towels over students' raised legs; students pull the sides of the towel to curl up their bodies.

Oblique Muscles (see Figure 4.21): The muscles alongside the rectus abdominis are strengthened by curling the body toward the opposite knee. Variations include crossing arms over chest and raising and lowering to the opposite side; resting the ankle on top of the bent knee, and, with fingertips behind the head, lifting elbow toward opposite knee (see Figure 4.22).

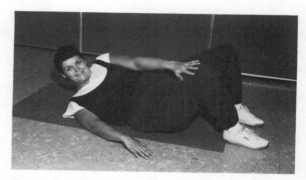

Figure 4.21   Curling up for the obliques

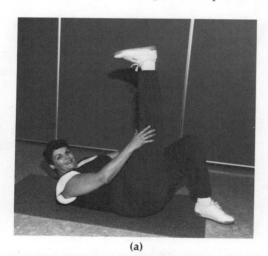

(a)

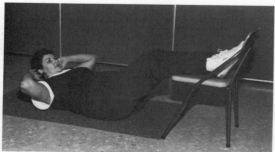

Figure 4.20   Curling-up for the rectus abdominis (b)

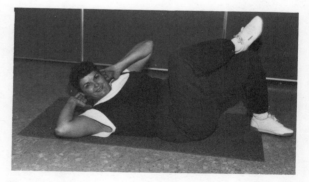

Figure 4.22   Variation for strengthening obliques

Transversus Abdominis Muscles: This is the deepest abdominal muscle, which encloses the lower fibers of the rectus abdominis. The transversus also activates with sit-ups and curl-ups, but more of its muscle fibers can be activated through such exercises as bicycle kicks, scissor kicks, and pike sits, all of which are quite difficult for overweight and obese individuals. When exercising the muscles of the lower abdominal area in full-figured individuals, use caution in your technique. Avoid placing undue strain on the lower back.

The safest, most effective hand position is hands under hips for back support. After a few weeks of regular exercise, I increase the level of difficulty by suggesting that students raise their head, as this causes the rectus abdominis muscles to contract and strengthen.

Muscle-developing exercises for the lower abdominals include the following: flutter kicks; raising and lowering legs from a bent-knee position; scissor kicks (legs should be 75 to 90 degrees from floor); and alternating presses outward, leading with the heel of the foot.

Some students are more comfortable resting on their elbows, which is an acceptable alternative to the fully reclining position. But since many students will have large busts in addition to large abdomens, exercising from a slightly propped position can be extremely uncomfortable, as a great deal of pressure is exerted on the chest and diaphragm.

Pressure-Relieving Exercises Following Abdominal Routines. After the abdominal series, you will want to lead exercises to stretch out backs and tummies. A simple exercise that FFFers enjoy is simply pressing their lower back into the mat in a bent-knee position (see Figure 4.23). Hold for several seconds, repeat two or three times. Another favorite stretch is demonstrated in Figure 4.24. Extend both arms and legs and stretch slowly to the right, then slowly to the left; repeat three times on each side.

Hips and Outer Thighs (Abductors)

In each hip and thigh exercise, as the participant lies on her side, leg muscles are maintained in a contracted position and seldom raised more than 45 degrees from the floor to avoid swinging the leg upward. Exercises require continuous muscle control and fluid movement. The proper form is knees slightly bent, feet flexed, head either propped on hand or resting on upper arm. An easy beginner's exercise requires students simply to raise and lower the top leg, with the knee bent. Begin with one set of eight repetitions, and two routines per side. Within three to four weeks two more routines should be added per side, to a maximum of four. Lead the class through a brief stretch after each exercise. After a few weeks of classes, stretches will be necessary only after each exercise series.

One of the most effective exercises for FFF hips and thighs is a slow leg lift (see Figure 4.25), with the top leg held at a 45-degree angle from the body. For a variation, bring the knee up toward the abdomen, foot flexed, then push (or press) the leg out to the front of the body (see Figure 4.26). Watch carefully that students aren't swinging or kicking their leg out from the knee, but rather pushing from the upper thigh outward.

Standard leg lifts are appropriate to FFF members as long as the movements are smaller and con-

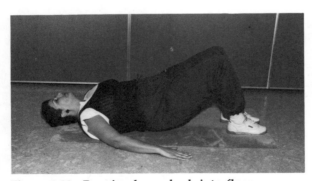

Figure 4.23   Pressing lower back into floor

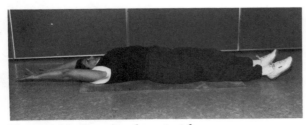

Figure 4.24   Favorite class stretch

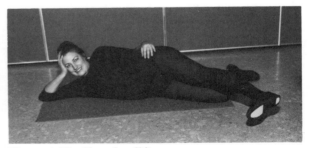

Figure 4.25   Slow leg lift

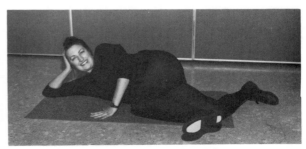

Figure 4.26   Variation of slow leg lift

centrated. To avoid overworking the hip tensors, the toes of the top leg should point toward the floor, and the student should be leaning forward slightly.

Inner Thighs (Adductors)

Full Figure Fitness exercises designed to strengthen the inner thighs are similar to conventional inner-thigh exercises, but the lifts are slower and the feet should remain flexed for hip and knee stability. Students can rest on one side, bottom leg extended with instep toward ceiling, opposite leg with knee bent and foot flat on floor. From this position the class can perform lower leg lifts, pushing (never kicking) the bottom leg outward, and leading with the heel, alternately bending and extending the bottom leg from a raised position. After each leg series, relieve tightness in the muscles by stretching the inner thighs.

Buttocks and Hamstrings

Proper body alignment is important for this series. The preferred position is resting on forearms and knees, a precaution against lumbar strain. Hands and knees position is acceptable for outer thigh exercises, because the leg is held out to the side, thus avoiding pressure to the back.

Once again, routine exercises such as those demonstrated in Figures 4.27 and 4.28 are appropriate, but, as always, the movements should be small and concentrated. If you are leading an extended leg lift exercise, avoid bringing the foot down to the floor. Instead, press the leg gently, or lift and lower no more than 12 inches from the starting position. This will keep muscles contracted while avoiding thrusting movements from floor to ceiling, which can put a lot of pressure on the spine. Variations include drawing the letter L with the leg (lift, lower, squeeze in, bring out); perform-

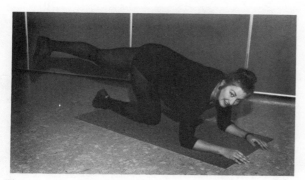

Figure 4.27 Fanny firmer

ing heel presses away from the body (start with knee slightly bent, then extend leg fully and push out, as shown in Figure 4.29); and bending knee, extending leg (again, lead with the heel—the knee will bend farther here than in the preceding exercise).

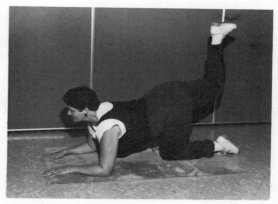

Figure 4.28 Fanny firmer

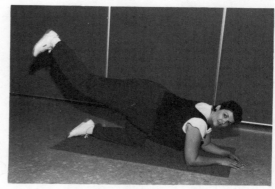

Figure 4.29 Variation of fanny firmer

Adductor muscles can also be strengthened from this position: Hold the leg out and squeeze it in toward the opposite leg. Individuals whose knee problems preclude positions on their knees can perform this exercise on their side, with their lower leg bent slightly. The extended top leg squeezes down toward the lower leg. The *squeezing* movement contracts the adductor muscles, so be sure that students aren't simply raising and lowering the leg from this position, or swinging their leg side to side from the forearms and knees position.

From this same position, release tension by bringing the buttocks toward the heels and sliding arms forward. The mad cat stretch is another excellent stretch following this exercise series: From hands and knees position, begin by lowering head, arching back up toward ceiling as you pull in hips and abdominals. Reverse the position by raising the head, lowering the back, and pushing the seat out.

Quadricep Muscles

To exercise the quadricep muscles, assume a seated position, one leg extended, the other foot flat on floor with knee bent (see Figure 4.30). Lean back on hands (or elbows, whichever is more comfortable). Raise and lower the leg. Variations are: knee in, leg out, raise and lower the leg (in, out, lift, and lower), knee in, leg out; extend leg and draw squares, circles, or the letter *L*.

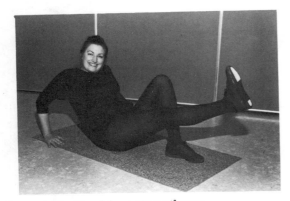

Figure 4.30   Quadricep strengthener

These exercises also strengthen the hip flexor muscles. A few students complain of groin pain within weeks of beginning exercises, and I think they may be overexerting during these particular exercises. (Once in a while I suffer such groin pain myself; usually during quadricep exercises.) With proper care, the pain usually goes away within a few weeks. Recommend ice and gentle stretches to students who have discomfort.

Waist and Arms

To improve muscle tone in the waistline (the internal and external oblique muscles), the arms play a role in helping stretch and move from side to side. By incorporating additional arm movements into the waist series, you can firm up many of the torso muscles as well.

Have your students sit up, with shoulders back and stomach tight. Legs should be positioned comfortably (straddled, curled under, or extended). The seated position makes it easier to isolate the working muscles by avoiding the tendency to push off the floor while standing during side bends. Students desiring a more demanding work load should use one- to three-pound weights, depending on their progress and conditioning.

Conventional arm and waist exercises are appropriate as long as they remain fluid and moderately paced: hands at ears, elbows out, bend side to side; arms extended out, twist arms as you bend from side to side; punch up alternately toward the ceiling to the center directly in front, and side to side; pull an imaginary rope from the ceiling (a few of my cutups insist that one day a good-looking man is going to appear at the end of that rope and it'll all be worth it). Additional exercises to insert into this series are bicep and tricep exercises (bent-arm elbow squeezes with fists up; arms up, down, out, in; and so on).

Variations

Every now and then the instructor should alter the routine order so that students don't get into a rut. Wall exercises can be performed either after the warm-up (you're already there!) or on returning from the break. Many of the large muscle groups can be strengthened using the wall as your exercise prop.

Wall push-ups are effective for strengthening tricep and pectoral muscles. The position of the hands should be changed to include different arm muscles. For example, begin with hands against the wall, chest level, fingertips pointed up. After

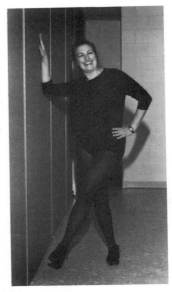

Figure 4.31   Inner thigh squeeze

one or two sets of 10 repetitions, let students bend forward, palms flat against the wall, to stretch out. Next, turn fingertips toward each other, perform 10 to 20 more reps, and stretch. Lastly (and they'll be moaning plenty by now), for those who can take it, point fingers away from each other and have at it again! Stretch and hold.

Hips, thighs, and buttock muscles can be exercised from the wall. Figure 4.31 demonstrates an inner thigh squeeze (again, the movement is slow and controlled); Figure 4.32 is a hamstring press (toe grazes the floor, leg presses backward). As the class improves its coordination, encourage them to try some of the exercises without using the wall for support.

To increase safety and efficacy, practice different exercises at the wall yourself before leading them in front of a class.

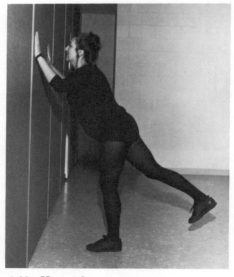

Figure 4.32 Hamstring press

Cool-Down—TGIF (Thank God I'm Finished!)

After a hearty workout everyone appreciates a few minutes to unwind with slow, delicious stretches, and deep, abdominal breaths. The cool-down is an integral part of the FFF program. Stretching and relaxing go hand in hand, and after a hot, sweaty workout, nothing feels better than kicking back and letting go.

The instructor's voice should reflect the mood of the music—calm and soothing. The cool-down

position is supine, knees bent, feet flat on floor, arms at sides.

Body scanning (a mental inspection to pinpoint tense muscles and let them relax) is helpful before beginning the stretches. Begin by scanning the muscles from the scalp downward. Take a minute or so to talk your students through the various muscle groups ("Now relax the muscles in your jaw, your neck, shoulders," and so on). Ask them to pay particular attention to the eyebrows, jaw, and shoulders. If there's tension in those muscles, there's probably tension elsewhere in the body.

After they've scanned down to the tips of their toes, relax further by taking full, deep breaths through the nose and blowing out gently through the mouth. When breathing deeply, the abdomen rises and lowers, not the chest or shoulders. Students may need to practice deep abdominal breathing, since it is often the opposite of their accustomed method of breathing.

Begin the stretches with slow neck stretches (side to side), followed by shoulder shrugs up toward the ears. Slide arms overhead and stretch up. Repeat some of the abdominal stretches, such as back presses into the mat and others. Draw one knee up, extend the opposite leg, alternate. Hip rolls also feel comfortable after exercise.

Stretch hamstring muscles by raising one leg, grasping the thigh (knee unlocked) and gently pulling the leg toward you. Slowly point the toe, then flex the foot to stretch the calf muscles. A recommended back stretch (Figure 4.33) is accomplished by drawing a knee toward the abdomen and pulling the leg gently towards the head while extending the opposite leg. Hold for several seconds. Alternate.

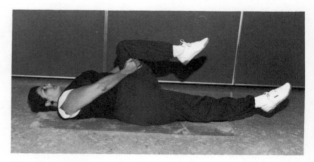

Figure 4.33 Back stretch

Continue deep breathing exercises. Tell the class to completely let go and R-E-L-A-X. Remind them that they must *allow* their bodies to relax or stretch—they can't force it. This is a good time to recheck pulses so that students can observe their rate of return to normal. The lower the pulse, the better.

Next, ask students to assume a seated position by turning to the side and propping themselves up (this is the preferred method for overweight adults to rise from a supine position). Follow the guidelines for seated stretches after the break. Because your students' body temperatures may still be rising, it is unwise to ask them to stand up immediately from a supine position. They could become dizzy, or even faint. A couple of minutes of seated stretches reduces the likelihood of postexercise light-headedness.

Lastly, stand up and roll the shoulders back several times. (Exercises that squeeze shoulders back are preferable to ones that round shoulders out. Stooping and lifting are a feature of daily ac-

tivities, while the opposing movement is not.) Stretch the right arm to the ceiling, then the left arm. Stretch over to the side, and then forward. Lace fingertips together at the back and try to raise arms while squeezing shoulder blades together (do not roll forward toward the floor).

Applause, Applause

At the end of class, thank the students for coming, and ask that they give themselves a round of applause for their efforts. Your words of encouragement will inspire them to make the Full Figure Fitness program an integral part of their lives!

Chapter

5

FFF—FYI
Instructor's Concerns

Regular exercise has the same benefits for overweight bodies as it does for lean ones—except that the external changes might not be as readily apparent. According to experts, "Exercise may carry important benefits for the overweight person even in the absence of weight loss. In sufficient amounts, physical activity can ameliorate nearly every ill consequence of obesity" (Greenwood, 1983, p. 49). Many of the beneficial changes will, of course, depend on the individual's commitment to weight control and exercise. Like everybody else, overweight people have moments of tremendous motivation and remarkable willpower, followed by periods of indulgence and lack of inspiration. Unfortunately, a fat person's motivation to exercise can be difficult to sustain. A talented instructor can help stimulate the desire to exercise by continually making comparisons between life before exercise and life after exercise—both from a physiological and a psychological perspective. Remind your students how much better they *feel* when they exercise. Assure them that although regular exercise may not make us thin, it most assuredly prevents us from getting fatter!

Benefits of Regular Aerobic Exercise

The following section describes the most significant changes produced in overweight men and women during a period of regular physical activity. Of course, there are many other advantages accompanying FFF exercise that readers can look forward to discovering in their own programs.

Reduced Blood Pressure and Improved Circulation

As you have seen in previous chapters, because of the stress placed by excess fat on the cardiovascular system, obese individuals are often in higher risk categories for heart and vascular ailments. The benefit of improved circulation is therefore highly significant for this group. The tissue that makes up our vital organs requires a constant supply of oxygenated blood. If the blood flow becomes diminished because of plaque buildup, the arteries lose elasticity, weaken, and become rigid. They can no longer expand and contract with the pulsing flow of blood. Eventually, worn arterial walls can become completely clogged and rendered useless. The result can be stroke, heart attack, or kidney failure.

Through regular, sustained aerobic exercise (20 minutes or more at least three times weekly), blood flow improves throughout the body. The heart muscle is strengthened, and resting heart rate (which is a barometer of a healthy, or healthier, heart) is gradually lowered.

Increased cardiovascular efficiency due to increased activity has had a profound effect on resting heart rate and blood pressure in a significant number of FFF participants. After twelve to sixteen weeks of regular attendance, about 30 percent of the hypertensive students have had their blood pressure medication reduced or eliminated. A few who had been taking several medications for a host of maladies were gradually weaned off one or more. In one case, the only remaining "prescription" was "keep exercising"!

An interesting improvement relating (although perhaps indirectly) to circulation occurred recently with one of my students. I can't explain the phenomenon from a medical perspective, but I think it's worth mentioning. This particular student was a middle-aged woman with approximately 36 percent body fat, based on a body fat analysis she herself had requested. During a class break she showed me a hard mass, about the size of a quarter, just underneath the surface of her upper forearm. She said that at one time these lumps had practically covered her arms.

Her doctor had advised her that these were "fat masses" (medically referred to as lipedema, which is the accumulation of excess fat and fluid in subcutaneous tissues) and there was no way to get rid of them. Yet, on this day, I could feel no lumps besides the one. She explained that since she'd begun exercising, the masses had been gradually disappearing (lipoatrophy). Though I am only guessing, it seems logical that if the masses were once larger and greater in number, they must have been exerting some kind of pressure against her blood vessels. The fact that they seemed to be dissipating or disappearing would suggest, perhaps, an accompanying improved blood flow. In any event, the reduction of these fat globules was clearly a healthier circumstance than their existence.

Incidentally, this particular student has recently been taken off her antihypertensive, diuretic, and antidepressant medications. She says that her systolic blood pressure is normal, and her diastolic blood pressure is several points below average. As her physical well-being improved, she began to take command of her life once again. Today, with doctor's approval, the only pills she swallows are vitamins. Interestingly, this is the same student whose husband enrolled her in the program, drove her to the facility, and practically dragged her into the class before she felt ready to take that first step toward self-help.

I think it is safe to assume that your own FFF students can look forward to similar results. The benefits of physical fitness far exceed the loss of a few pounds. The following study supports the same effects of exercise on overweight people that have been achieved by many in the FFF program.

In 1978, in Sweden, Per Bjorntorp and his colleagues found that a six-month exercise program consistently lowered blood pressure in twenty-seven overweight women. These women did not lose significant body fat during their activities. The evidence (and my own experience supports this) suggests that hypertensive individuals who have been unsuccessful at long-term weight loss may be able to improve their condition with exercise (cited in Bennett & Gurin, 1982).

Many researchers believe that exercise, and where necessary weight loss, may be reasonable alternatives to prescription medications that often have adverse effects, are expensive, and may have long-term health risks.

Improved Self-Concept

Being fat in a weight-conscious society can undermine self-esteem (see "Stress and Disease" in chapter 2). Yet some studies have shown that overweight men and women in physical training programs exhibit marked improvement in self-satisfaction, self-acceptance, and a sense of personal worth (Hanson & Neede, 1974). A Harris poll in 1979 found that physically active people reported more self-confidence, a better self-image, and greater psychological well-being than inactive people.

Most of my students have expressed a renewed sense of control after a period of regular activity, which facilitates their ability to resolve problems of personal dissatisfaction and poor body image. Psychologist Judith B. Elman (1986) states that "control over one's life—the ability to make choices—is vital for a positive self-image and a feeling of personal power."

Another member of the program, a director of a mental health clinic, has described her own improved mental health after participating in an uninhibited class where she was free to laugh, chat, and "let it all hang out." She said the emotional outlet was as important for her as the physical one. This woman gets a kick out of my own occasional whining about exercising. (I sometimes indulge in a bellyache over the ceaseless need for continuous exercise—or else!) I haven't met anyone who gets goose-pimply in anticipation of a grueling workout. Students have more fun when their teacher joins in a group "sufferalong!"

Exercise may be easier to adopt on a long-term basis than continuous or sporadic attempts to reduce food intake. The benefits of exercise offset its difficulties. The body adapts to the demands of physical exertion by increasing muscular strength and endurance, whereas long periods of food restriction produce diminishing returns, and increase both physical and psychological stress.

During periods of increased stress, feelings of lethargy often result with the release of adrenaline and cortisol, both stress-related hormones. These hormones are metabolized by exercise, which decreases their undesired effect. Endurance activities result in the secretion of endorphins by the brain. These small, morphine-like substances can produce a feeling of exhilaration, which reduces stress and, through a complex process, may even reduce fat storage.

In a conscientious program of regular exercise, the health benefits are lasting. The discipline of a good workout makes people feel better about themselves. This improved self-concept may be instrumental in the development of long-term lifestyle changes that lead to permanent weight control and a healthier life.

Increased Metabolism

Not only does the metabolic rate increase during exercise, but the effects of exercise keep the metabolism elevated for several hours afterward. Thus more calories are burned, making the body even more fuel efficient. During the hours after exercise the metabolic rate is about 10 percent higher than before exercise. The postexercise period *alone* can account for a weight loss of five or ten pounds in a year.

Appetite Control

We have already seen that exercise is effective in lowering insulin levels in obese individuals, which helps control hunger drives. Exercise increases the responsiveness of the cells to insulin, thereby discouraging the overproduction of insulin (see chapter 2, "Diabetes").

Researchers have also shown that, for obese people in particular, aerobic exercise of moderate intensity does not increase appetite. In fact, hormones secreted during exercise actually reduce appetite, and these hormones rise to higher levels in obese individuals than in lean individuals. The findings suggest that exercise is more likely to stimulate appetite in lean individuals than it is in obese ones (Geliebter, 1982).

Because aerobic exercise uses primarily fat for fuel, an aerobic program of long duration (more than twenty minutes) and at moderate intensity (65 to 85 percent of maximum heart rate) may be more effective at reducing food intake than high intensity, short-term, anaerobic exercise, according to Swenson and Conlee's 1979 study (cited in Wolman, 1982). The anaerobic process (known as glycolysis) converts glucose into lactate or pyruvate, which results in short-term energy (only seconds in duration) in the form of ATP in the muscles. Aerobic activity may, in fact, be most effective when it occurs shortly before the usual mealtime. A 1978 study by Epstein and colleagues found that when students exercised just before their lunch period, they ate less than when they exercised at other times. This is more than likely due to the redistribution of blood flow—more blood is pumped into working muscles during physical activity.

Improved Lipoprotein Ratios

Exercise may also increase the ratio of beneficial high density lipoprotein (HDL) to destructive low density lipoprotein (LDL). Lipoproteins are surplus cholesterol, which is a kind of blood fat found in animal products (never in plants). Most of the body's supply of cholesterol is synthesized in the liver, but some of it—sometimes too much of it—is absorbed from the diet.

Simply stated, there are two kinds of cholesterol. HDL, the beneficial variety, is made up of abrasive, scavenger protein molecules, which function to remove fat and cholesterol from the inside surface of the arteries and carry them into the liver for excretion. LDL, the destructive variety, consists of large, sticky globules. It is responsible for the accumulation of cholesterol levels in the blood. LDL can become imbedded in the artery walls, forming a fatty-fibrotic lesion called *atherosclerotic plaque*, which narrows the arteries and impedes blood flow, increasing the risk of heart attack. A high level of blood, or serum, cholesterol is an even more serious health hazard than high blood pressure.

Weight Loss

Weight loss through exercise alone tends to be very slow (approximately 1 pound per week). However, slow, consistent weight loss is far more beneficial than the quick or irregular variety. Slow weight loss through exercise represents the loss of body fat, not of muscle. If the increase in activity is sustained, the weight will not likely return, which prevents the body from suffering the damaging effects produced by recurring weight fluctuations.

A study by William Zuti and Larry Golding (1976) suggests that the combination of exercise and reduced food intake produces more significant fat loss and lean tissue gain than diet or exercise alone. In this study, 25 women were randomly assigned to one of three regimens: diet alone, exercise alone, or a combination of diet and exercise. The diet group reduced their intake by 500 calories per day; the exercise group expended 500 calories during each one-hour session; the combination group reduced calories by 250 and increased energy expenditure by 250. The difference in pounds lost was not statistically significant: 11.7 for dieters, 10.6 for exercisers, and 12.0 for those who combined the two. However, only the combination group significantly increased their lean body, or muscle, mass.

Weight loss is not always evidence of physical conditioning. It may be an added benefit, but should not be established as an FFF goal. Members do not typically lose weight during the first several weeks of class. Some lose little weight but increase their muscle mass and improve their

physical appearance through the redistribution of the weight that is there.

Exercise and Extreme Obesity—When Nothing Seems to Work

Sadly, there is a small fraction of students for whom exercise does not seem to elicit discernible change. Such people are usually extremely obese (often referred to as "morbidly" obese by medical professionals, though such terminology is inappropriate for the instructor's use in class).

Certain physicians and psychologists who work with extremely obese patients are of the opinion that this condition is permanent. Massive weight loss can be achieved through semistarvation, but it is rarely lasting. I know of many former clients of weight loss centers who lost between 50 and 100 pounds, only to regain it all within a year or two. There comes a point with various diseases and disorders when the damage cannot be reversed; obesity exceeding levels of 50 percent of normal body fat appears to be one of them.

Special Considerations for the FFF Participant

Our students are initially unaccustomed to continuous activity. In the early weeks of the program they tire easily and complain of aches, pains, and exhaustion. Sustained movement of one's own body weight, for some, is strenuous and difficult, and instructors must work hard to motivate individuals to keep moving. The stress of excess body weight unsupported by strong muscle tissue can cause increased incidence of hip, knee, and ankle problems.

This section focuses on special problems that will eventually have to be addressed in FFF classes. Should the fitness leader encounter situations not mentioned here, she will need to rely on her own experience, training, and research to guide her. Class leaders will need to review each health history form carefully, and discuss any concerns with the student. Medical problems unfamiliar to you should be discussed with the patient's physician. Alternative movements and body positions should be reviewed before beginning the exercises to reduce the individual's chance of discomfort later on. Additionally, it is always a good idea to have several chairs around the exercise area for students who will need to rest.

Physical Limitations and Restrictions— Forewarned is Forearmed!

The first session of FFF will be your most difficult session. The program will be unfamiliar to your students, and will present issues and possibilities beyond those of conventional fitness programs. Fat people often have an extreme resistance against exercise—usually more so than against restrictive dieting. Their inactivity is a preferred state. Psychiatrist Hilde Bruch (1973) notes that "It is much harder to induce a fat person to walk an extra step than make him refrain from eating an extra bite. He will do so if bullied and strictly supervised or constantly encouraged" (p. 314). True enough. So as forewarned instructors you must be forearmed as well. Be prepared to teach your students the relevance of exercise to *their lives*. Once you've determined that your participants understand why exercise is so important, tell them again! Bully (in good fun)! Supervise! Constantly encourage!

During this first session, some participants will evidence various conditions and maladies related to their size and inactivity. This section will help you (and them) prepare for some of the problems that might evolve as they begin to move muscles that have lain dormant for a long time.

Arthritis in the Hip Joints. Physicians often recommend exercise to their patients with arthritis. Exercise helps prevent joint atrophy and keeps surrounding muscle tissue viable. However, depending on the severity of the problem, some individuals may find aerobic movements uncomfortable to sustain. If pain (not discomfort) during exercise does not subside after a few weeks, the participant might be advised to partake in a non-weight-bearing activity such as swimming or water exercise.

Students with problems of the hip area should be alerted to the importance of maintaining body alignment, particularly of the hips, knees, and feet. Overweight people often suffer from iliotibial band syndrome (see "Warm-Up," chapter 4). Correct stretches and body alignment will reduce the likelihood of the problem occurring during exercise.

Bad Knees. Pain felt at, or on the sides of, the knee is a familiar complaint among overweight in-

dividuals. In such cases, aerobic activity isn't always as painful when the patella (the kneecap) is stabilized laterally. This can sometimes be accomplished by the use of a ''horseshoe'' knee brace to be worn during class on physician's approval. Patients can request a prescription for the brace so that the cost (about forty dollars) can be covered by insurance.

Lateral movements during aerobic exercise occasionally cause knee discomfort to the afflicted students. Rather than shift their bodies from side to side, students should be instructed to turn 45 degrees and step forward in the direction of the movement. Steps such as the grapevine or carioca, requiring lateral cross steps, can also produce soreness. As an alternative, students can either step side to side without the cross steps, or simply step or march in place during any movements that place undue stress on the knee.

Knee pain might prevent these students from comfortably performing exercises (such as doggies or hydrants) on hands and knees. Demonstrate alternative exercises performed lying on the side. For example, hydrants can be executed on the side by keeping the upper knee bent while raising and lowering the leg. Rear leg lifts would require raising the top leg slightly and gently pressing it back.

Weak Ankles. The strain of a large body that is unaccustomed to frequent movement produces ankle discomfort for a few FFFers during aerobic exercise. For these individuals, too, body alignment is essential for reducing strain on ligaments and joints. Exercises such as ankle rotation and plantar and dorsiflexion will help strengthen this area, as will low-impact aerobic exercise that increases the size and strength of lower leg muscles.

Leg Cramps. Several students have complained of leg cramps during low-impact activity or while walking for prolonged periods. Poor circulation may be the cause of this cramping, which occurs when (a) the muscle undergoes prolonged contraction, or (b) the blood flow to working muscles becomes inadequate. Oxygen supply in the blood is reduced and may be insufficient to meet the muscle's requirements during exercise. The result is immobilizing cramps or pain while walking. In most people, this affliction (called intermittent claudication) is self-inflicted—the result of poor health habits. The most effective treatment is to modify these habits. Exercise is strongly recommended because of increased blood flow through vasodilation.

During aerobic exercise or walking, students who suffer leg cramps should stop briefly and rest. Usually the pain subsides quickly, and they can resume activity. If the pain is prolonged, have them sit down and prop up their feet. If the pain is severe and/or lasting, they should consult their physician. Marked reduction of leg cramps usually occurs within 6 to 12 weeks of regular exercise.

Inner Thigh Burns. Inner thigh burns are a common occurrence in overweight people, but the problem is exacerbated by the continuous movements during the cardiovascular phase of exercise. Constant leg friction during exercise can cause discomfort and rashing. Recommend petroleum jelly to your students to soothe irritated skin. Leotards, knee length shorts, or jog pants should be worn to reduce chafing.

Foot and Leg Relief: The Correct Aerobic Shoe. Even low-impact aerobic activity warrants the purchase of a shoe built for shock absorption, stability, and comfort. This is especially true for exercisers whose shoes will need to accommodate the stresses of a large body. Old, worn-out sneakers do nothing for weak ankles and aching legs.

Students suffering from weak ankles might try a midcut, or hightop, aerobic shoe for added support. Recurrent problems of the hips, knees, or ankles require the expertise of a podiatrist to determine whether the problem is a correctable structural defect.

Proper Flooring

Although FFF involves low-impact aerobics, the type of floor used in the workout is important because the burden of excess body fat can be stressful to joints during movement. Individuals with arthritis, particularly of the hips and knees, will suffer the effects of improper flooring much more than other participants. Hardwood flooring such as on basketball courts is best. The least desirable is concrete (or linoleum over concrete) because the impact of movement is absorbed by the lower extremities. Remember, even in low-impact aerobics the force of the landing is still 1.5 to 2 times that of body weight.

The Effect of HBP Medication on Target Heart Rates

High blood pressure medication slows down the exercise heart rate. Therefore, pulse rates of individuals on antihypertensive drugs will be slower and not an accurate representation of actual physical exertion. For example, the average pulse rate during FFF aerobics is between 20 and 23 beats using a 10-second count (120 and 138 bpm, respectively). Students on antihypertensives average between 14 and 19 beats (84 and 114, respectively), depending on the strength of the medication.

In these cases, participants should check pulses to note any irregularities, but they will also need to gauge their activity levels by "listening" to their bodies (perceived exertion). If they feel sweaty but not drenched, breathy but not breathless, and exhilarated but slightly "spent," they are exercising aerobically. The "talk test" is helpful in familiarizing students with appropriate exercise exertion. If they have enough oxygen to talk to the person next to them, but not enough to hold a note or sing, they are exercising within their target heart range.

Who Qualifies for the FFF Program?

It would be awkward to employ any weight restriction in this program. There are many variables to be considered when assessing body size (somatotype, percent body fat, bone structure, etc.). Participants should be allowed to decide for themselves whether FFF meets their needs. It is important, however, to retain the focus on exercise for the full-figured individual, rather than on low-impact aerobic exercise. This will discourage anyone from joining who simply prefers that type of workout to the other varieties. Being fat is a unique condition—hold "outsiders" to a minimum.

Aerobic Jargon—Impossible Dreams

Because overweight people have special physical limitations not always understood by the rest of us, certain phrases common to conventional fitness programs are inappropriate to this one. During the aerobic phase, for instance, a common low-impact step call is "elbow to opposite knee." Some of your students can't even see their knees from a standing position, let alone reach one with an elbow! It is more suitable to call out "elbow *toward* opposite knee," at least during the first few sessions.

The phrase "knee to chest" should be avoided for the same reason—the tummy plays interference. Substitute "knee lift" or "raise your knee." I remember the first time I called out "knee to chest," back in the days of my Full Figure inexperience. Somebody from the back row hollered out, "She's gotta be kidding!" and the class had a hearty laugh at my naivete.

Abdominal curls involve another standard exercise call—"chin to chest"—when students attempt to lift the head and shoulder to contract abdominal muscles. If they have extra "chins" the first one won't reach their chest. They will raise and lower their heads with noses pointed straight up to the ceiling. The substitute call in a supine position is "raise your head." (The call from an erect position, such as during neck stretches, is simply "lower your head.")

Deceiving Appearances.   A sidenote might be appropriate here regarding what might appear to be a lack of cooperation from some of your people during abdominal exercise. When your students perform abdominal curls, it might look as though the larger among them are barely moving. Although they may be working their abdominal muscles arduously with the simple raising and lowering of their heads, the movement will be almost imperceptible until some of the interfering "fleshy folds" are reduced. If, on careful observation, you see that the student's shoulders have risen slightly off the mat, rest assured that this small movement will contract abdominal muscles. Repeated attempts at curl-ups will eventually result in more discernible movement and tighter muscles.

Do-able Demos.   Your demonstrations should provide a practicable example of the exercise, so demonstrate only at the skill level that most of your students can realistically imitate. Bring your elbow *toward* your knee, not to it. Curl up as far as you expect the students to curl. Stretch as far as most of them can stretch. Anything more could produce envy and discouragement ("I'll never be able to do that, so why bother?").

Fat Terminology.   Fat people know they are fat, so it is unreasonable to avoid use of the word in a program where the subject comes up constantly. Phrases such as "abdominal fat," or "if you have too much fat on your..." are perfectly acceptable. As long as the words "fat, obese, and overweight" are used objectively, and not critically or insensitively, there's no problem. Remarks such as "Let's work on those fat thighs!" however, might get you a "fat" lip!

Impersonal Pronouns.   Fitness instructors have become accustomed to hearing body parts referred to as "that" and "those," and carry on the tradition in their own classes. But terminology that sounds normal to you and me may sound dehumanizing to the layperson. I admit that this is my personal bias, but please refer to "those" parts as "your" parts, since the parts make up a whole person, and "that" person deserves respect!

Use of the Comfort Index

Under the direction of my exercise advisor, Deb Knight, I developed the Comfort Index (see Figure 5.1) for two reasons. The first was to provide the student with a heightened sensitivity to the subtle changes elicited by exercise. Many of us pay little attention to the fruits of our exercise labors beyond weight loss. A color chart such as this will delineate their more far-reaching advantages.

Second, the Comfort Index helps the instructor ascertain the effectiveness of the exercises. Students will occasionally suffer in silence rather than complain to an instructor that some of the exercises hurt. This sheet provides instant feedback so that the exercises can be finely tuned to the specifications of your students.

During the first 8 weeks of the first session, indexes should be distributed weekly or biweekly; as students progress, monthly distribution will suffice. Provide one red and one blue pencil to each student. Instruct them to color in blue that portion or portions of the body that feel improved with exercise. Areas of the body that feel strained or sore with exercise should be colored in red. Color *all* relevant areas of the body. Ask that students focus on behavioral changes as well as physical ones. If they feel less stressed, color the head blue; if they can suddenly walk up a flight of stairs without being winded, they should color the chest area blue.

Collect each sheet and ask participants if they had any interesting revelations they'd like to share. Take no more than 5 minutes to discuss their responses, unless their insights are especially informative.

On reviewing each page, be particularly aware of the red colors. More than a couple of red lower backs could mean that you need to modify some of your abdominal exercises, or perhaps you are bouncing during aerobics and they are following your lead. Remember that students will imitate whatever you demonstrate during class.

Medical Considerations

As stated in chapter 3 (see "Legal Liability") all participants are required to complete a health his-

COMFORT INDEX

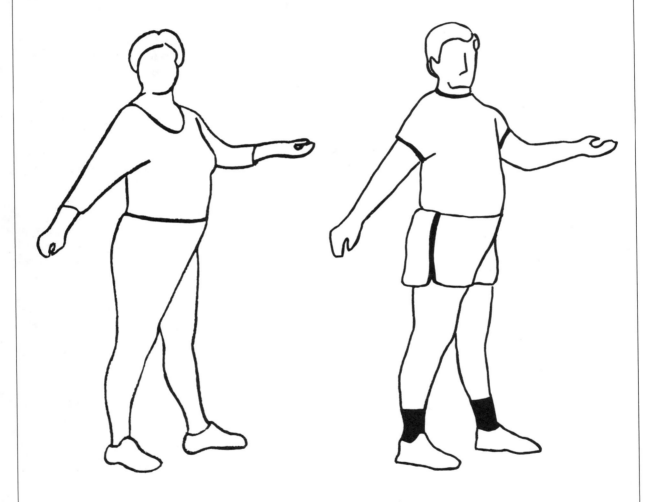

- Color sore areas in red.
- Color areas that have improved with exercise in blue.

Figure 5.1 Sample outlines of comfort indices. Have participants color sore areas in red. Color areas that have improved with exercise in blue.

tory. Review each form carefully before admitting anyone into the program. Questions regarding the medical profile should be discussed with the individual's physician. As you learned in chapter 2 (''Health Risks''), blood pressure screening is necessary, and physician's authorization may be required in cases of untreated hypertension or any other health matters that may concern the instructor.

fitter people without having to become thin people. *If the potential instructor cannot accept permanent overweight as a fact of life for some, he or she will not be effective in conducting a program of this nature.* Obese individuals, like members of other minorities, view themselves through the eyes of others. Our participants must be accepted by the instructor without condition.

The Qualified Full Figure Fitness Leader

The FFF instructor lays the groundwork for the success or failure of the program. If he or she demonstrates responsibility, enthusiasm, understanding, and talent, the program will be off to a successful start. If he or she is inexperienced, apathetic, disorganized, or unmotivated, the program will quickly develop a bad reputation, and any attempts to begin anew may be fruitless. It is, therefore, essential that the FFF leader be the very best candidate for the job.

FFF leaders must be certified in both CPR (cardiopulmonary resuscitation) and first aid and should hold at least one certification as a fitness leader (as offered by International Dance-Exercise Association [IDEA], Aerobic Fitness Association of America [AFAA], or other established fitness organizations, the YMCA of the USA, or the American College of Sports Medicine). The ideal candidate should also have at least one year's experience as a fitness instructor.

Outstanding fitness leaders are invariably voracious readers in the areas of exercise, sportsmedicine, and the health sciences. Research in exercise physiology is ongoing, and new information occasionally renders generally accepted theories obsolete. The serious fitness instructor has a hearty appetite for knowledge about the industry.

Continuing education can be obtained through the many leadership and fitness workshops available to professional fitness employees. By joining one of the previously named organizations, he or she can remain informed about upcoming workshops in the area, as each organization generates a mailing list for this purpose.

Lastly, and if all of the above qualifications are met, the qualified FFF leader must agree with the premise of this book—that fat people *can* become

Humor and the Fitness Leader: Wisecracking Workouts

A hearty sense of humor is an invaluable asset for the FFF leader. As previously mentioned, members are often highly stressed and look to this program to relieve some of their tensions. FFF breaks through their isolation and draws out uninhibited participation. One hour of rowdy exercise interspersed with comic relief leaves the group feeling lighthearted and looking forward to the next class. Raucous laughter has generated business for my own program—one of my regulars first joined because she'd often heard our laughter from down the hall, and just had to find out what was so funny!

When students are comfortable with their instructor, they are less restrained in their movements. (Timidity in an exercise class makes for a lousy workout!) When they can loosen their controls, a marvelous time will be had by all. And the students will invariably provide the instructor with some delightful entertainment of their own. I wish I had a nickel for every one-line repartee I've heard delivered in my classes. Like the time I sort of lost count when executing leg lifts. I cajoled the group that after the last set there was only ''one more leg to lift!'' To which a student soberly replied, ''Right, Bon—yours!''

Providing Nutritional Information

Because so many participants are interested in diet, a special section on nutrition is offered here as background information only—FFF is not intended to be a weight reduction program. However, my overweight students so frequently request information about proper diet and nutrition that expert advice may be helpful to the instructor. When answering questions, FFF instructors should make clear that they are passing along the advice of experts and are not themselves qualified nutritional counselors.

This information was prepared especially for the Full Figure Fitness program by members of the Southern Ohio Health Services Network. Many thanks to registered dietician Monica Alles-White, MS, RD; to Ginni Mohrfield, MS, RD; to Lisa Ford, MS, RD; and to Amy Czajkowski, MS RD, for their efforts in preparing this insightful material on nutrition as it applies to an overweight population.

Nutrition Principles

Nutrition is simply the relationship between diet (what we eat and drink), nutrients, and health. The food and drink we consume are classified into four basic food groups: milk, meat, fruits and vegetables, and breads and cereals. There exists another food group of "undesirables"—or those foods that are high in fat and sugar and low in nutrients.

The essential purpose of eating is to obtain the necessary calories, nutrients, and fiber to sustain life. Our calories, containing our energy source, come from three of the six essential nutrients—carbohydrates, protein, and fats. Carbohydrates, sugars, and starches derived from plants and animals should contribute at least half of our total daily caloric intake, as they are the body's chief source of fuel.

The next most important source of calories is protein, which is necessary for growth, tissue maintenance, protection against disease, and production of hormones and enzymes. For adults, the recommended dietary allowance of protein is .8 grams per kilogram of desirable body weight, or roughly 20 percent of daily caloric intake. More protein is required during growth and pregnancy.

Last in the category of essential nutrients is fats. Yes, our bodies do require fat for survival, though not necessarily in mass quantities! Fats aid in the absorption of vitamins A, D, E, and K. They are also an important energy source (aerobic activity primarily uses fat for fuel) and should comprise about 30% of our total calorie intake. When attempting weight loss, however, fat is the single most important nutrient to decrease in the diet because of its high caloric value (9 calories per gram

compared to 4 calories per gram in carbohydrate and protein).

The other three essential nutrients—vitamins, minerals, and water—assist in metabolism and other important body functions. Although alcohol does provide energy (7 calories per gram), it is

Table 5.1   Low-Calorie Basic-Four Food Plan

Milk—2 Servings Daily
    1 serving = 1 cup fluid skim, low-fat, or 2% milk
           1 cup buttermilk made from skim milk
           1/3 cup nonfat dry milk
           1½ ounce low-fat or part skim milk cheeses
           1½ cup low-fat cottage cheese
           1 cup plain, unflavored low-fat yogurt

Meat and Meat Alternatives—2 Servings Daily
    1 serving = 3-4 ounces lean beef and pork cuts
           2 eggs
           3-4 ounces poultry, turkey, or chicken
           3-4 ounces fish
           1 cup cooked dried beans and peas
           1 cup tofu
           (avoid lunchmeats, sausages, and frankfurters)

Bread, Cereal, and Grains—4 Servings Daily
    1 serving = 1 slice whole grain bread
           1 roll or biscuit
           ½ cup cooked unsweetened cereal
           ¾ cup unsweetened cold cereal
           ½ cup rice
           ½ cup macaroni or noodles
           4 saltines

Fruits and Vegetables—4 Servings Daily
    1 serving = ½ cup unsweetened fruit or vegetable juice
           1-2" diameter fresh fruit
           ½ cup unsweetened canned fruit
           ½ cup cooked vegetable
           1 cup raw vegetable

Fats and Oils—Not Less Than Two Tablespoons Each Day

Miscellaneous Foods—As Diet Allows
    Best bets are: Sugar-free gelatin, pudding, and chewing gum
           Angel food cake
           Ice milk, sherbet, and fruit ices
           Diet soft drinks

numbered among the "undesirables" because of its lack of nutrients.

For the most part, all foods contain one or more of these nutrients, in varying amounts. Milk and milk products contain carbohydrates, protein, fat, calcium, vitamins A and D, riboflavin, and phosphorus. Meats and meat alternatives provide protein, fat, iron, thiamin, niacin, and riboflavin. Fruits have carbohydrates, fiber, and depending on the type of fruit, varying amounts of vitamins A and C and potassium.

Vegetables give us small amounts of protein, in addition to carbohydrates, vitamins A and C, potassium, and fiber. Whole grains, breads, and cereals contain our chief source of carbohydrates, protein, fiber, iron, thiamin, and B-vitamins.

When an individual consumes more of these nutrients than his body's energy output requires, he may become overweight. Yet this condition can often be avoided by sensible food choices from the basic four food groups (see Table 5.1 for low-calorie basic-four food plan).

Fiber

Fiber is an essential part of our diets because it is beneficial in preventing colon cancer, treating diverticulosis, controlling blood sugar, and relieving constipation. Foods that contain fiber are usually high in complex carbohydrates and low in fat. Furthermore, high-fiber foods require more chewing, fill the stomach, and take longer to digest than refined foods. Hence the individual feels satisfied for longer periods of time. For this reason, a diet for weight loss should contain foods high in fiber to enhance eating pleasure and satiety.

Fiber is found in fruits, vegetables, grains, and legumes. There are two types of fiber: water soluble, such as that found in oatmeal, beans, citrus fruits, and apples; and water insoluble, such as bran fiber. Fiber content in foods is based on *dietary* fiber; processing and cooking food can decrease fiber content.

Water

Because our bodies are made up of 50 to 65 percent water, with daily losses occurring through respiration, perspiration, and waste, it is easy to understand why water is necessary to live. In order to prevent dehydration and constipation, we must replace these losses continuously. During exercise, for example, we should consume two cups of fluid for every pound of weight lost. If we do not replace fluid in our systems, dehydration can develop, which affects electrolyte balance and/or initiates chronic constipation. Water is the preferred fluid to replace what our body loses because it is readily absorbed by the tissues.

When the body obtains the necessary amount of water for optimal functioning, all sorts of healthy things happen: Fluid retention is alleviated, endocrine gland function improves, and more fat is burned, or used as fuel, because the liver is then free to metabolize stored fat into usable energy. All are excellent reasons to consume at least eight 8-ounce glasses of water a day; and even more when exercising briskly, when the weather is hot and dry, or when one is overweight.

Energy Expenditure

Two factors affect an individual's daily energy or calorie requirement: basal metabolic rate (BMR) and physical activity. The factors that influence BMR are (a) body composition, or the ratio of muscle tissue to adipose tissue; (b) endocrine glands secreting hormones and thus regulating metabolic rate; (c) nutritional status, which is described as either well nourished or undernourished; (d) sleep; (e) fever or illness; (f) muscle tonus; and (g) pregnancy.

Basal metabolic rate is lower if large proportions of adipose, or fat, tissue are present. It is also slowed down in conditions of underweight, starvation, during sleep, and in cases of decreased secretion of the hormone thyroxine by the thyroid gland. Factors that increase BMR are aerobic exercise, tensed muscle tonus (the slight, continuous contraction of a muscle), pregnancy, fever, and illness.

Concerning the second factor influencing energy requirements, physical activity, the degree and type of exercise will dictate the amount of calories required. The combination of BMR and physical activity dictates the number of calories burned from food and drink.

Exercise increases caloric expenditure. In addition, aerobic exercise elevates BMR for several hours following an exercise period. During aerobic exercise at the target heart rate, the body uses fat as its predominant energy source, and improves the cardiovascular system at levels between 60 and 85 percent of maximum HR.

Social and Medical Influences

Because eating is often a social affair, social support is an essential component of a weight reduction program. Support, or the lack thereof, from family, friends, co-workers, and peers, can influence one's ability to stick with a program. An individual who feels frustrated will often eat her way through the anxiety.

Existing medical conditions may also influence weight reduction. It is therefore important to consult a physician *before* seeking professional assistance to help you lose weight. When "all systems are go," the registered dietician can develop a specialized diet plan that will meet nutrient needs and help the individual achieve and maintain the desired weight.

Weight Management

Any successful weight management plan should begin with a realistic goal, an assessment of energy needs, and a personalized, flexible diet plan. Restrictive diets that severely limit caloric intake, or that omit any of the basic food groups, are counterproductive and should be avoided. (Appendix E contains some handouts you may want to share with your participants.) An appropriate calorie-restricted diet in conjunction with regular exercise is the desired approach to weight reduction.

A balanced diet that utilizes the basic four food groups provides the essential nutrients at a caloric level that relies upon fat stores to meet energy demands (see Table 5.1). It is useful to remember that no single food is "fattening" and no single food is capable of "burning calories." Each gram of carbohydrate and protein contributes four calories of energy, while each gram of fat contributes nine calories. One pound of body fat is equal to about 3,500 calories. Therefore, daily restriction of 500 calories below total calories required to maintain weight will promote the loss of one pound per week (500 × 7 days = 3,500). Weight loss of one to two pounds per week is recommended in a sensible, realistic diet plan.

Behavior Modification

Weight loss is challenging at best, discouraging and depressing at worst. Anyone who makes the decision to lose weight should possess a positive attitude and should be capable of realistic goal setting. If nutritional habits have been sorely lacking, a complete turnabout in establishing new eating habits may be necessary. Such changes are best

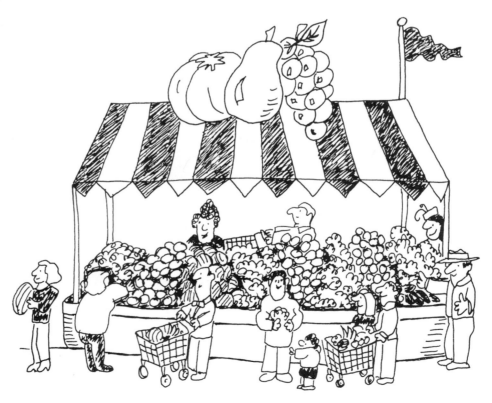

engendered and enforced under the direction of a caring professional.

The following are some suggestions from nutrition professionals, which may be of help to FFF students who inquire about weight reduction:

- Plan meals in advance; plan snacks, special occasions, weekends, and holidays.
- Bake, broil, roast, boil, or stew, because these cooking methods do not use additional fats. Trim all visible fat off meat before cooking. Avoid heavy sauces and gravies because they are usually high in fat.
- Avoid sampling while cooking.
- Avoid eating alone.
- Decide to eat in one room, sitting down.
- Measure all foods to be sure to control calories. Avoid serving family style because second helpings are too accessible.
- Use smaller plates to create the impression of more food.
- Eat slowly. Enjoy the texture, appearance, and aroma of each food.
- Minimize leftovers. For example, freeze food in the correct, measured portions.
- Avoid skipping meals.
- Prepare raw vegetables to keep in the refrigerator for snacks.
- Shop from a list and stick to it.
- Don't shop while hungry or tired.
- Avoid buying low-nutrient or high-calorie foods.
- Shop with a limited amount of money. This should help to avoid buying extra food.
- If you eat extra calories or food not in your diet, don't abandon your plan. Resolve to follow it with the very next meal.
- Finally, reward yourself with a special activity, event, or small gift.

In addition, nutrition education for the overweight individual should include information on moderating salt intake, reducing the amount of refined carbohydrates, altering the balance of unsaturated (plant) fats and saturated (animal) fats, eating regular balanced meals, and ensuring that sensible eating habits are developed and maintained.

Summary

Today's consumers have an assortment of edibles and beverages that would have caused our ancestors terrible confusion ("No kidding! 20th century man really eats those weird looking items from a paper sack, and rinses them down with an effervescent syrup from an aluminum cylinder? Gross!").

Some nutritionists believe that we have too many available foods of unacceptable nutritional quality. Yet these very foods are the staple of an increasing number of American diets. Many different things influence our food choice and eating habits. Once poor nutritional habits are developed, improving them can be quite a challenge, as the rewards of positive lifestyle changes are not achieved overnight. It is remarkably simpler to instill healthy habits at an early age, so that reform need never be an issue.

Questions Commonly Asked by Health Care Professionals and Fitness Instructors About Full Figure Fitness

Question. Why should our facility offer FFF when we have beginner fitness?

Answer. Overweight people do not want to exercise with people who are not overweight, regardless of their fitness level. Furthermore, beginner programs are often progressive, becoming more difficult as the weeks pass. If the overweight person observes classmates advancing rapidly to higher levels and new programs, he or she may become intimidated, and will be less enthusiastic about his or her own progress. However, if a beginner class remains at a very low level, overweight students will be discouraged from reaching their full potential because, unlike the others, it is unlikely that they will want to "advance" to aerobic workouts at a later date, and may, therefore remain unchallenged in a beginner program.

FFF is a moderate-level program that provides a challenging, fun workout for beginners as well as for "lifetime members."

Question. Do you recommend a mirrored exercise studio to help students monitor their form?

Answer. Not unless such a studio is the only available space. Overweight people have a poor body image, so it is unlikely they would want to watch themselves exercise. The mirrors might be distracting; participants might feel uncomfortable surrounded by them. The FFF experience should be positive in every aspect. Students should be made as comfortable and secure about themselves as possible. A three-way look at their bodies as they move about a room could produce discouragement and disappointment in themselves. Let's leave 'reality therapy' to professional counselors.

Question. How much do you charge for this program?

Answer. The many responsibilities involved in developing and maintaining a quality program merit a higher fee for FFF than for conventional programs. Achievement-oriented instructors who are knowledgeable, aggressive, and professional command decent wages. They'll spend time planning, organizing, and marketing, as well as consulting with physicians about various medical concerns. If the instructor receives higher wages for the demands of the job, the cost of the program should be proportionately higher.

Question. Should FFF be offered in conjunction with a weight control program?

Answer. Since the focus of FFF is exercise and fitness education performed in a nonjudgmental atmosphere, an auxiliary program of any variety is contradictory. It denies that fitness alone is a worthwhile goal for overweights.

Certainly, programs providing nutritional information and reasonable weight control guidelines have merit for us all. But I think it's prudent to offer them to the public in general rather than to associate them with the FFF program.

Question. Isn't water exercise preferable for obese people?

Answer. Water exercise and other non-weight-bearing activities are beneficial to almost everyone. Buoyancy reduces stress to the joints. Many FFF students enjoy water exercise programs as well. However, some participants are reluctant to be seen publicly in a bathing suit. Others prefer the high energy and increased caloric expenditure generated in aerobic fitness programs.

With a few modifications, FFF can be easily transformed into a water exercise program. For example, aerobic steps would remain about the same, only slower. Floor work would be replaced with exercises against the shallow edge of the pool. A standing cool-down would close the hour.

If you wish to pursue a water exercise FFF, consult with an aquatics director about appropriate modifications.

Question. Do you encourage wrist and ankle weights as students progress?

Answer. One-pound wrist weights are useful for students wishing to increase the intensity of their workout. Stronger students wear one-pound weights during low-impact aerobics, and two- to three-pound weights during arm and waistline exercises.

However, my exercise consultant advises that ankle weights, though fine for physical therapy, are not recommended for fitness training. They can place undue stress on the knees and lower legs during aerobics. They are particularly troublesome to knees during inner thigh strengthening exercises, when the leg is turned and the instep faces the ceiling. If you compare the human leg to the branch of a tree, you can see how adding weight to its weakest and narrowest point can cause problems.

Question. What kind of workout clothes should students wear? Instructors?

Answer. Bright, colorful clothing should be encouraged. Students look and feel better in cheerful colors, but poor body image prevents some of them from wearing anything that makes them stand out. The problem of low self-esteem can be addressed indirectly by complimenting students who come to class dressed "cheerily."

Though students are invited to wear leotards if they like, I'd encourage instructors to wear something less revealing. Need I detail the disheartening effect of a svelte beauty (or "hunk") in skintight apparel admonishing a group of fat people to "lift those legs!"

Program Evaluations

Program evaluations are useful in assessing both the successes and the shortcomings of your program. A sample evaluation is provided here for you to use at the end of your session.

Evaluations should be kept anonymous to guarantee uninhibited honesty. People who are put in the position of rating others (especially those they like) are usually very generous in their analyses of their performance. Although flattery is nice, it isn't always productive. Ask your participants to be brutally honest. Don't collect the evaluations yourself, but let participants place them in a folder as added protection against "intimidated flattery." Use the feedback you receive on your evaluation to make modifications in your program.

Full Figure Fitness
Program Evaluation

Location _____ Instructor _____

....

1. Overall evaluation of this program: (circle appropriate number)
   very dissatisfied   1   2   3   4   5   6   7   8   9   10   very satisfied

2. How much impact did this program have on you?
   no impact   1   2   3   4   5   6   7   8   9   10   great impact

3. Did the instructor address the needs of the class?
   not at all   1   2   3   4   5   6   7   8   9   10   very much

4. The class experience was:
   unpleasant   1   2   3   4   5   6   7   8   9   10   very pleasant

5. General impression of classroom facility:
   very dissatisfied   1   2   3   4   5   6   7   8   9   10   very satisfied

6. do you feel better after participating in this program?
   not at all   1   2   3   4   5   6   7   8   9   10   very much

7. Has your participation in this program increased your knowledge of fitness?
   not at all   1   2   3   4   5   6   7   8   9   10   very much

....

Please let us know:

8. What you liked most about the program _____

   _____

   _____

9. What you liked least about the program _____

   _____

   _____

10. Recommendations for improving the program _____

    _____

    _____

11. Do you plan to participate in another Full Figure Fitness class? (Please explain your answer)

    _____

    _____

    _____

Epilogue

Most people like to know that, in the course of their lives, they've made a worthwhile contribution to the world. But few ever have the opportunity to engender dynamic lifestyle changes in others. Fitness instructors and health care professionals are fortunate in that we enjoy regular reminders that our efforts on behalf of someone else have paid off. If a sense of achievement and pride in accomplishment had dollar values, FFF instructors could take an early retirement.

When a man finds out that his blood pressure has gone from 165/100 to 120/80, and he can see his toes pointing out from under him for the first time in years, he's going to share his good news with the person who paved his way.

When a woman suddenly has the energy to handle all of her responsibilities, and enough left over to bake cookies, she'll seek out the person who gave her the impetus to make changes.

Someone who has remained isolated and alone because she felt like nobody gave a hoot is going to have a good word for the person who pulled her out of her rut and back into the land of the living.

These are healthy lifestyle changes that the Full Figure Fitness instructor can look forward to. She'll meet people who will begin her program feeling depressed and angry. Then she'll watch them transform into laughing, vital people once again.

The Full Figure Fitness program is only an instrument—the instructor will be the driving force that makes it work. He or she can spark the fire of determination in people whose own sense of value has been lost through years of neglect.

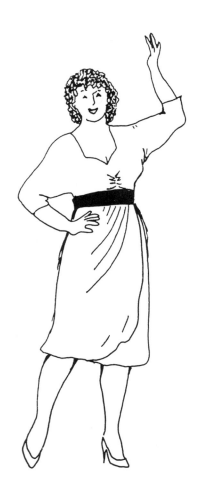

Appendix

A

Sample Flyers to Advertise Your Program

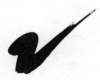

Full
Figure
Fitness

Developed by author and fitness specialist Bonnie D. Kingsbury, *Full Figure Fitness* is designed to meet the fitness needs of overweight adults **safely, effectively,** and **enjoyably.**

The Full Figure Fitness program will improve each important component of your fitness (cardiorespiratory, flexibility, muscular strength and endurance, and percent body fat). In addition, you will enhance your fitness education and appreciation through informative printed material. Motivational instruction is provided by an experienced, certified fitness leader.

Inactivity breeds physical and psychological stress —

Fitness feels better —
It looks better —
It is better!

And now it is attainable for YOU! So take that first step toward a **healthier, happier life.** You'll be glad you did!

At last! A realistic, comprehensive fitness program for overweight men and women.

Now you can improve your physical conditioning and work off stress in the company of others who share similar needs and concerns.

*If you are overweight,
and
you've had enough*

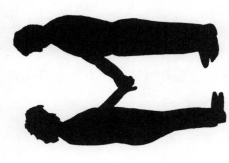

- Dieting
- Depression
- Lethargy
- Bad Advice

*and you are searching for
something better . . .*

*For information,
call or contact:*

Full Figure Fitness

FINALLY—AN EFFECTIVE AND REALISTIC EXERCISE PROGRAM

DESIGNED ESPECIALLY FOR INDIVIDUALS

WHO ARE OVERWEIGHT AND OUT OF CONDITION

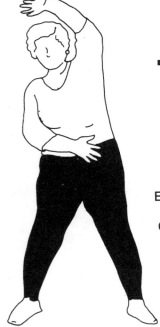

Our certified instructor will help
CHARGE UP YOUR MOTIVATION through

SAFE, easy-to-follow exercises;

EDUCATION and instructional materials in fitness and nutrition;

CARDIOVASCULAR conditioning through low-impact aerobics;

RELAXATION techniques;
AND MUCH MORE!!

Now you can enjoy a complete fitness program in the company of others who share your needs and concerns.

Come in and talk to us (or give us a call) and let us help you obtain RESULTS THAT LAST AND LAST!

Figure A.1 Sample outlines to aid in making easy advertisements for your programs.

Big Men's Workout

FINALLY—AN EFFECTIVE AND REALISTIC EXERCISE PROGRAM

DESIGNED ESPECIALLY FOR INDIVIDUALS

WHO ARE OVERWEIGHT AND OUT OF CONDITION

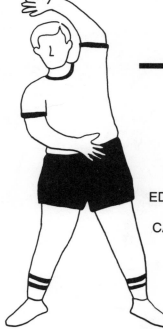

Our certified instructor will help
CHARGE UP YOUR MOTIVATION through

SAFE, easy-to-follow exercises;

EDUCATION and instructional materials in fitness and nutrition;

CARDIOVASCULAR conditioning through low-impact aerobics;

RELAXATION techniques;
AND MUCH MORE!!

Now you can enjoy a complete fitness program in the company of others who share your needs and concerns.

Come in and talk to us (or give us a call) and let us help you obtain RESULTS THAT LAST AND LAST!

Appendix
B
Full Figure Fitness
Participant Forms

Full Figure Fitness
Waiver, Release,
and Indemnity Agreement

In consideration of permitting me, _____,
to participate in the following described activity: _____
beginning on the _____ day of _____, 19____,
I HEREBY VOLUNTARILY RELEASE, DISCHARGE, WAIVE, AND RELINQUISH any and all
actions or causes of action for personal injury, property damage, or wrongful death occurring to
me arising as a result of engaging or receiving instructions in said activity or any activities incidental
thereto wherever or however the same may occur and for whatever period said activities or instructions may continue. I, for myself, my heirs, executors, administrators, and assigns, hereby RELEASE,
WAIVE, DISCHARGE, AND RELINQUISH any action or causes of action, aforesaid, which may
hereafter arise for me or my estate, and agree that under no circumstances will I or my heirs, executors, administrators, and assigns prosecute, present any claim for personal injury, property damage,
or wrongful death against _____ (institution), its facilities,
or any of its members, officers, instructors, agents, employees, for any of said causes of action,
whether the same shall arise by the negligence of any said persons, or otherwise. IT IS MY INTEN-
TION BY THIS INSTRUMENT TO EXEMPT AND RELIEVE _____ (institution),
its members, officers, instructors, agents, and employees FROM LIABILITY FOR PERSONAL
INJURY, PROPERTY DAMAGE, OR WRONGFUL DEATH CAUSED BY NEGLIGENCE.

I, for myself, my heirs, executors, administrators, and assigns agree that in the event any claim for
personal injury, property damage, or wrongful death shall be prosecuted against _____
_____ (institution), or its members, officers, instructors, employees, or agents,
I SHALL INDEMNIFY AND SAVE THEM HARMLESS OF, from and for any and all claims or causes
of action by whomever, whenever, or wherever made or presented for personal injuries, property
damage, or wrongful death.

I acknowledge that I have read the foregoing and have been fully and complete advised of the
potential danger incidental to engaging or receiving instruction in the activity described hereinabove
and am fully aware of the legal consequences of signing this instrument.

Dated this _____ day of _____, 19 ____

_____   _____
Witness   Signature of participant

Full Figure Fitness
Health History Form

Name _____ Age _____ Sex _____ Date _____

Address _____ Marital Status _____

Phone (Home) _____ (Business) _____ Zip _____

Birthdate _____ Height _____ Occupation _____

Personal Physician _____ Weight _____

Physician's address _____ Phone _____

_____ Zip _____

(Check if yes.)

PAST HISTORY:	FAMILY HISTORY:	HAVE YOU RECENTLY HAD?
Have you ever had?	Have relatives had?	
__ Rheumatic fever	__ Heart attack	__ Chest pains
__ Heart murmur	__ High blood pressure	__ Shortness of breath
__ High blood pressure	__ High cholesterol	__ Heart palpitations
__ Heart trouble	__ Diabetes	__ Cough on exertion
__ Disease of arteries	__ Congenital heart disease	__ Cough up blood
__ Varicose veins	__ Heart operations	__ Back pain
__ Lung disease	__ Other	__ Arthritis
__ Operations		__ Swollen legs
__ Injuries to back, knees, ankles	Explain _____	
__ Epilepsy	_____	
__ Diabetes		
__ Heart attack		
__ Other		

Risk Factors

SMOKING: Do you smoke cigarettes? _____

How many? _____ For how many years? _____

Age started? _____ When did you stop? _____ Why? _____

DIET: Current weight? _____ One year ago? _____ At 21? _____

Are you dieting? _____ Why? _____

EXERCISE: Do you exercise or engage in sports? _____ Which ones? _____

How often? _____ How far do you walk daily? _____

Is your job: _____ Sedentary? _____ Inactive? _____ Active? _____ Heavy work?

Do you have discomfort, shortness of breath, or pain when exercising? _____

_____ Specify _____

MEDICATION: Are you currently taking oral contraceptives? _____

Are you taking other medication? _____ Which ones and what are they treating?

_____

_____

BLOOD PRESSURE _____ RESTING HEART RATE _____

Full Figure Fitness Application and Medical Clearance Form

I hereby make application to enroll in the Full Figure Fitness course and I (please check appropriate response):

_____am 35 years of age or older and request medical clearance from my physician.

_____am less than 35 years of age and I have no known history or symptoms of coronary artery disease and I request to be admitted without medical clearance. I understand that the instructor reserves the right to require medical clearance before admitting me to fitness classes.

_____am less than 35 years of age and request medical clearance from my physician.

Signature of applicant _____ Date _____

Applicant's name _____
(please print)   (First)   (Middle initial)   (Last)

Applicant's street address _____

City _____ State _____ Zip_____

Telephone (Business) _____ (Home) _____

Employed by _____ Position _____

- -

For the physician:

I have examined the above applicant and approve of his/her participation in a program of physical exercise. Any limitations are noted below. (Please print or type.)

Limitations _____

_____

_____

Physician's name (Please print) _____

Physician's street address _____

City _____ State _____ Zip_____

Telephone (Office) _____ (Home) _____

Signature of physician _____ Date _____

Appendix
C
Welcome to the Program

Congratulations—you've made the decision to improve the condition of your body! During the next weeks you'll have much to look forward to: You'll meet new people, learn about fitness and health, increase muscular strength and endurance, make your heart more efficient, increase your supply of oxygen, and learn how to simply relax and let go.

Full Figure Fitness is not choreographed—all you have to do is follow the bouncing instructor. Initially, you may feel a few reminders that your muscles have been on holiday. They may resent your effort to return them to the work force. Don't despair—a little discomfort is normal, and very soon you'll feel brighter and more energetic than you have in a long time.

Before beginning, it will be helpful to read the following tricks of the trade:

1. Never work through pain. Mild discomfort is expected from time to time, but pain is a warning to STOP.
2. If you start to feel dizzy or weak, rest until the feeling passes.
3. Pace yourself without worrying about anyone else. Everyone is too busy working to notice if you stop for a break. We're in this

to get fit—competition isn't part of the format.
4. Drink water before, during, and after class. Your muscles are comprised of 70-75 percent water. In addition, as your body adapts to the stress of regular exercise, you will begin to perspire freely and you'll need water to keep your system in balance.
5. Never hold your breath while working out. Exhale on the exertion, and keep breaths slow and relaxed. This will send a signal to the working muscles not to tighten so that the exercise is easier and more effective.
6. Send your bathroom scale on a six-week cruise to the Dead Sea: Exercise builds muscle (don't worry, you won't end up looking like Arnold Schwarzenegger), and muscle is heavier than fat. You may actually gain pounds during the first few weeks— but those pounds represent muscle and water weight—not fat. Scientists have found that sometimes a person will lose fat for as long as two weeks without losing a pound of weight, thus your scale cannot tell you the full story. (Scales are notorious liars anyway!)
7. Protein is essential in maintaining the body's water balance. If it is inadequate, extra water

may be drawn into tissues, producing puffiness and swelling. Some people who think they are overweight may actually be waterlogged due to poor nutrition and (yes, it's true) insufficient fluid in the system.

8. Outside of class, look for exercise opportunities. Use stairs instead of escalators and elevators. Save time driving around the parking lot looking for a space—park far away and walk the extra paces to your destination. Stretch your body! Stretching (never bouncing) increases the blood and oxygen supply to your muscles.

9. Exercise does wonderful things for the body and mind, but not always for the hips. Weight loss with exercise alone is very slow—usually one pound per week. But that is permanent loss of fat, not muscle. The pounds won't creep back up your thighs when you're not looking. Research shows that weight loss of more than two pounds per week is almost always temporary. Slow weight loss is usually permanent and, because the individual is exercising, he or she is shedding only fat weight, not muscle.

Our goal in Full Figure Fitness is to get fit and feel terrific. If weight loss occurs, that's okay. If it does not, that's okay too.

10. Exercise is NOT fun—but IT IS funny. Some of the situations we get into provide wonderful laughs, especially when the class is ROWDY. So come on, YELL, WHOOP, and HOLLER! Full Figure Fitness is SASSY and FUNKY—get ready to LOOSEN YOUR CONTROLS!

Appendix

D

Calculating and Monitoring the Exercise Heart Rate

Monitoring the Exercise Heart Rate

Step 1: Calculating Your Heart Rate

Teach participants to calculate their training heart rate range at the first or second meeting. If you do so at an orientation meeting, you can save your-self class time. Prepare handouts of the formula presented here and use posters to reinforce your points.

The following is a commonly used formula (Karvonen's) for calculating a training heart rate for normal, healthy adults. (The right-hand column provides explanations for each number or variable.)

220

A constant value in the formula, representing the heart's anatomical and physiological limits.

minus *age* (years)

Remember that age (along with other factors) influences the heart rate. The maximal heart rate starts to decline progressively at about age 25. The decline is estimated to occur at the rate of 1 beat per year.

minus *resting heart rate*

Due at least in part to individual differences in levels of fitness, resting heart rates will vary. The multiplied by 60 and 90 percent (.6) and (.9)

best time to take your resting heart rate is the first thing in the morning before getting out of bed. Participants taking medication should check with their physicians concerning possible effects of the medication on resting and exercise heart rates. Some medications commonly used for high blood pressure will lower the heart rate.

To stress the cardiorespiratory system, you should work out somewhere between 60 to 90 percent of your maximum heart rate reserve. The American College of Sports Medicine recommends using 60 to 90 percent of the maximum heart rate reserve (Fox, 1979) for healthy adults.

plus *resting heart rate*

Due to the variations in participants' resting heart rates, this value is taken into consideration.

ANSWER:
HEART RATE TARGET RANGE

These numbers are your training heart rate range. When performing aerobic activities, participants should strive to work out within this range because it represents a pace that is sufficient for achieving cardiorespiratory training benefits and that can be maintained easily. For example, if you stay within this range, you should be able to work out for 20 to 30 minutes continually, whereas if you exceed this range, you may fatigue after only 10 to 15 minutes. The lower end of the range is a safe range for beginners, while more advanced participants can work out at the upper end.

To determine a training heart rate range for a beginning-level 20-year-old woman who has a rest-

ing heart rate of 74 bpm, at 60 and 90 percent maximum you would calculate as follows:

$$
\begin{array}{r}
220 \text{ (Max HR)} \\
- 20 \text{ (Age)} \\
\hline
200 \\
- 74 \text{ (Resting HR)} \\
\hline
126 \\
\times .6 \text{ (\% Max HRR)} \\
\hline
75.6 \\
+ 74.00 \text{ (Resting HR)} \\
\hline
149.60
\end{array}
$$

$$
\begin{array}{r}
220 \text{ (Max HR)} \\
- 20 \text{ (Age)} \\
\hline
200 \\
- 74 \text{ (Resting HR)} \\
\hline
126 \\
\times .9 \text{ (\% Max HRR)} \\
\hline
113.4 \\
+ 74.00 \text{ (Resting HR)} \\
\hline
187.4
\end{array}
$$

Her exercise training range would be 150-187 bpm.

Step 2: Taking Your Heart Rate

Teach participants to locate their pulse and to count their heart rate. It is easy to find the pulse on the neck (either side of the Adam's apple). Follow your jawline until it ends and press lightly. Another convenient location is on the thumbside edge of the wrist (see Figure D.1). Major arteries surface close to the skin at these two sites, creating a strong beat.

Take the count with the index and middle fingers. When taking the pulse on the neck, be sure to apply only light pressure. Excessive pressure may cause the heart rate to slow down momentarily due to a reflexive action.

Have participants practice taking their heart rate a few times prior to the first workout. Establish cue words such as *heart check* to use when it is time for participants to take their heart rate. Insist on quiet during this time to facilitate accurate counting, but keep them *moving* rather than standing still. Stopping abruptly can cause blood to pool in the arms and legs and not return to the heart as efficiently as it should. The result can be light-headedness or even fainting. Select another cue word such as *go* and be sure that participants are counting *each* beat after the second you say go until the second you say ''stop.''

To get a minute count, first take a 6-second count and simply add a zero to the number of beats. You can also take a 15-second count and multiply this number by 4. The easiest method is the 6-second count, but the 15-second count is a little more accurate.

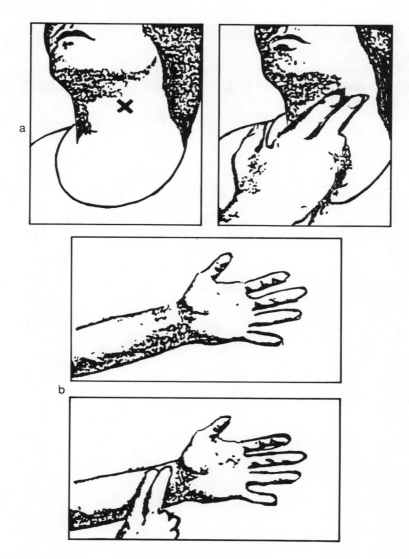

Figure D.1   Locations for taking the heart rate (a) the carotid pulse (b) the radial pulse

Step 3: Benefits of Staying in Your Range

Explain the benefits and importance of working out within the training range. The benefits are (a) you can be sure of getting just enough of a vigorous workout; (b) you won't fatigue as quickly should you continue to exceed this range; and (c) once you are familiar with working out within this range, you can gauge your participation in *any* aerobic activity.

Step 4: Making Adjustments

Teach participants how to raise and lower their heart rate by adjusting their performance during class. The heart rate increases when the movements/exercises involve both the upper and lower body. It also increases as the movements are performed in a more exaggerated manner, filling more space. That is, an individual who is working out below (not too common) his or her training heart rate can increase the intensity of the workout by, say, moving the arms as well as by doing the exercises more vigorously. An individual who is working out above his or her training range can do just the opposite—eliminate any unnecessary upper body movements and keep the movements smaller and closer to the body. Similarly, the intensity of locomotor skills (such as jogging) can easily be adjusted (to walking).

As participants continue to train, their resting heart rates will begin to decrease 6 to 8 weeks into the program due to adaptations of the cardiorespiratory system. Beginning participants' heart rates will rise quickly in response to exercise, but as they become more fit, they will have to work harder at attaining and maintaining their training heart rate.

Step 5: Using Visual Aids

Make posters of the heart rate formula and of locations for taking the heart rate. Include information about adjustments that can be made that affect the heart rate. Skillfully designed posters add color and brighten up the workout area. More importantly, posters help remind individuals of the points you've made about working out safely within the training heart rate range. Table D.1 represents calculated target heart rates.

Table D.1 Target Heart Rates

Age	Est. Max. HR	10-Second Count			Age	Est. Max. HR	10-Second Count		
		85%	70%	60%			85%	70%	60%
18	202	29	24	20	45	175	25	20	17
19	201	28	23	20	46	174	25	20	17
20	200	28	23	20	47	173	25	20	17
21	199	28	23	19	48	172	24	20	17
22	198	28	23	19	49	171	24	20	17
23	197	28	23	19	50	170	24	20	17
24	196	28	23	19	51	169	24	20	16
25	195	28	23	19	52	168	24	20	16
26	194	27	23	19	53	167	24	19	16
27	193	27	23	19	54	166	24	19	16
28	192	27	22	19	55	165	23	19	16
29	191	27	22	19	56	164	23	19	16
30	190	27	22	19	57	163	23	19	16
31	189	27	22	18	58	162	23	19	16
32	188	27	22	18	59	161	23	19	16
33	187	27	22	18	60	160	23	19	16
34	186	26	22	18	61	159	23	19	15
35	185	26	22	18	62	158	22	18	15
36	184	26	21	18	63	157	22	18	15
37	183	26	21	18	64	156	22	18	15
38	182	26	21	18	65	155	22	18	15
39	181	26	21	18	66	154	22	18	15
40	180	26	21	18	67	153	22	18	15
41	179	25	21	17	68	152	22	18	15
42	178	25	21	17	69	151	21	18	15
43	177	25	21	17	70	150	21	18	15
44	176	25	20	17					

Note. This table represents target heart rates for apparently healthy individuals only. If you are more than twenty pounds overweight or have a known heart condition, 60 percent of your maximum heart rate is recommended for your target area.

The DOs and DON'Ts OF EXERCISE

Demonstrating improper exercises can be more detrimental than not exercising at all. Memorize and teach your classes these dos and don'ts (Alter, 1983).

The DOs of Exercise:
Keep your body moving.
Provide your body with a balance of stretching and strengthening activity.
Feel the sensations of stretching and strengthening.
Stretch—

1. Hold the correct position for thirty seconds to a minute, or longer as necessary.
2. Actively feel the stretch in your muscles, not in your ligaments or joints.
3. Before and after any strengthening activity, stretch out the contracted muscles.

Strengthen—
1. Always protect your spine by putting your body parts in a safe, nonstraining position.
2. Do strengthening exercises slowly, moving the body part down and up against gravity.
3. When you are tired, do the strengthening exercise once more carefully.
4. Feel the exercise in your muscles, not in your joints or ligaments.
5. Guard against locking any joint.

The DON'Ts of Exercise:
Do not bounce.
Do not lock (hyperextend) your joints.
Do not arch your lower back or your neck.
Do not swing or do any exercise fast during warm-up or cool-down.
Do not "overbend" a joint.

Here is a list of common exercises *not* to do:
Do not do neck rolls.
Do not do shoulder stands.
Do not do fast arm swings during warm-up or cool-down.
Do not do waist twists.
Do not do back bends or back arching.
Do not do fast, straight-legged, arms-behind-head sit-ups.
Do not do toe touching with locked knees or with stomach relaxed.
Do not do deep knee bends.
Do not do "hurdler's sit" in an unsafe position.
Do not do "Japanese splits."
Do not do "triangle pose."

STOP ANY AND ALL EXERCISE IF IT HURTS.

Do trust your ability to distinguish between the safe feelings of stretch and the harmful feelings of pain.
Do take charge of your body, its health and well-being, by keeping in motion safely. Now you know what "safely" means.

Note. *From Surviving Exercise* (p. 109) by J. Alter, 1983, Boston: Houghton Mifflin Company. Reprinted with permission.

Appendix

E

Evaluating New Reducing Diets

New Diet or Exercise?

Ask yourself:

1. Is it controversial?
2. Are sensational claims being made, such as "no willpower needed," "eat all you want and still lose weight," "trim off inches of fat without exercise," and so on?
3. Is it based on little research, or research with animals rather than humans?
4. Is it a diet based on one group of foods or nutrients to the exclusion of others, or does it exclude one group of foods or nutrients?
5. Is the originator of the idea noted more for activity in an area other than health, nutrition, or exercise?
6. Does he or she seem more interested in media coverage than in the soundness of the program?
7. Are you required to purchase special foods, devices, books, or to take medications?
8. Is the promised weight loss rapid—more than two or three pounds a week?
9. Is its effectiveness supported only by user testimonials?

10. Has the program or concept been used widely for a number of years?
11. Does it make sense from everything you already know about diet and exercise?
12. Is it based on research that's been published in a peer-reviewed journal?
13. Are behavioral changes, as well as a means for controlling calories, suggested?
14. Is exercise suggested in conjunction with dietary changes?
15. Was the program conceived, and is it supervised, by qualified personnel with a medical/nutritional background?
16. Could you stick to the program for the rest of your life?

If you answer "yes" to questions 1-9, chances are you're hearing about the latest fitness fad. Think again before you spend money or risk your health on something that's not likely to work and may set back your fitness efforts. If you can answer "yes" to questions 10-16, you may be onto a real fitness classic, but check carefully that it's right for you.

From Diann Rivkin, RD, Nutricare

The Magical Weight Loss Myths

Have you heard the one about . . .
    . . . vinegar and grapefruit melting away fat?
    . . . protein not being fattening?
Yes? Then you have been myth-informed.
The Facts
    No food or pill can burn up fat.

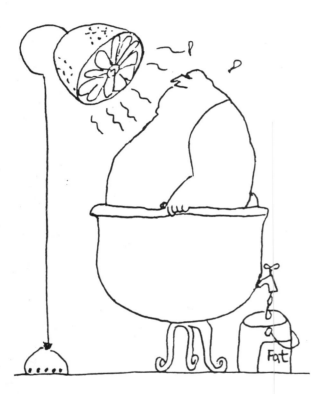

Nearly all foods (including foods with protein) have calories. Ounce for ounce, protein has as many calories as carbohydrates.

Many foods high in protein also contain fat. Fat supplies more than twice the amount of calories that protein and carbohydrates do.

Calories can be stored by your body as fat, whether they come from protein, carbohydrates, or fat.

The only way to lose weight is to make sure that the calories you consume from food and beverages are less than the calories you use for normal body functions and physical activity.

There are no miracles to losing weight. If you're thinking about trying a weight loss product or going on a diet, be cautious.

Some weight loss programs promise instant weight loss or claim you can eat as much as you want and still lose weight. These claims don't fit the facts.

Other plans require that you buy special pills, powders, or liquids and claim that they replace food or instantly melt away fat. Such fad diets may be easy to follow for a short time, but they are impossible to follow for normal, everyday eating. Any weight that is lost on these diets is probably regained quickly. The only thing that is permanently lost is your money.

Finally, many fad diets leave out foods from one or more of the basic four food groups. These diets are unhealthy since your body needs foods from all of the groups to get all fifty or so nutrients necessary for health.

From Diann Rivkin, RD, Nutricare

References and Suggested Readings

Books

Alter, J. (1983). *Surviving exercise*. Boston: Houghton Mifflin.

Beller, A.S. (1977). *Fat and thin: A natural history of obesity*. New York: Farrar, Straus, and Giroux.

Bennett, W., & Gurin, J. (1982). *The dieter's dilemma*. New York: Basic Books.

Bruch, H. (1973). *Eating disorders: Obesity, anorexia, and the person within*. New York: Basic Books.

Cannon, G., & Einzig, H. (1985). *Stop dieting because dieting makes you fat*. New York: Simon & Schuster.

Cleave, T.L. (1974). *The saccharine disease*. Bristol: John Wright and Sons.

DuCoffe, J., & Cohen, S. (1980). *Making it big*. New York: Simon & Schuster.

Epstein, L.H., Mosek, B., & Marshall, W. (1978). *Pre-lunch exercise and lunch-time caloric intake*. 1,15.

Geliebter, A. (1982). Exercise and obesity. In B. Wolman (Ed.), *Psychological aspects of obesity* (pp. 291-310). New York: Van Nostrand Reinhold.

Golding, L.A., Myers, C.R., & Sinning, W.E. (1982). *The Y's way to physical fitness*. Chicago: National Board of YMCA.

Greenwood, M.R.C. (Ed.). (1983). *Obesity: Contemporary nutrition*. New York: Churchill Livingstone.

Krause, M., & Mahan, K. (1984). *Food, nutrition and diet therapy: A textbook of nutritional care*. Philadelphia: W.B. Saunders.

Kuntzleman, C.T. (1975). *Activetics*. New York: Peter H. Wyden.

Kuntzleman, C.T., & Consumer Guide Editors. (1978). *Rating the exercises*. New York: William Morrow.

Louderback, L. (1970). *Fat power: Whatever you weigh is right*. New York: Hawthorn Books.

Mathews, D., & Fox, E.L. (1976). *The physiological basis of physical education and athletics*. Philadelphia: W.B. Saunders.

Mirkin, G. (1983). *Getting thin—All about fat*. Boston: Little, Brown.

National Research Council. (1980). *Recommended dietary allowances* (9th rev. ed.). Washington, DC: National Academy of Sciences.

Nygaard, G., & Boone, T. (1985). *Coaches' guide to sport law*. Champaign, IL: Human Kinetics.

Olds, R. (1984). *Big and beautiful*. Washington, DC: Acropolis Books.

Orbach, S. (1978). *Fat is a feminist issue*. New York:

Berkley Books.

Overeaters anonymous. (1980). Torrance: Overeaters Anonymous, Inc.

Pawlak, L. (1986). *The R.D. Leader of the fitness boom, exercise prescription.* (self-published)

Polivy, J., & Herman, C. (1983). *Breaking the diet habit.* New York: Basic Books.

Radar, W. (1981). *No diet program for permanent weight loss.* Los Angeles: J.P. Tarcher.

Remington, D., Fisher, G., & Parent, E. (1983). *How to lower your fat thermostat.* Provo: Vitality House International.

Rodin, J. (1982). Why the losing battle. In B. Wolman (Ed.), *Psychological aspects of obesity* (pp. 37-38). New York: Van Nostrand Reinhold.

Rosenzweig, S. (1982). *Sportsfitness for women.* New York: Harper and Row.

Wilmoth, S.K. (1986). *Leading aerobic dance exercise.* Champaign, IL: Human Kinetics.

Wolman, B.B. (Ed.). (1982). *Psychological aspects of obesity.* New York: Van Nostrand Reinhold.

Wood, P. (1983). *California diet.* Mountain View, CA: Anderson World Books.

Journals

Brownell, K. (1984). The psychology and physiology of obesity: Implications for screening and treatment. *Journal of the American Dietetic Association,* **84**(4), 406.

Cahnman, W.J. (1968). The stigma of obesity. *Sociological Quarterly,* **9**, 283-299.

Canning, H., & Mayer, J. (1966). Obesity—Its possible effect on college acceptance. *New England Journal of Medicine,* **275**, 1172-1174.

Elman, J.B. (1986). The loneliest of the long distance runners. *Runner's World,* **21**(7), 34-39.

Goldblatt, P.B., Moore, M.E., & Stunkard, A.J. (1965). Social factors in obesity. *Journal of the American Medical Association,* **192**, 1039-1044.

Hamburger, W.W. (1951). Emotional aspects of obesity. *Medical Clinics of North America,* **35**, 483-499.

Hanson, J.S., & Neede, W.H. (1974). Long-term physical training effect on sedentary females. *Journal of Applied Physiology,* **37**, 112-116.

Lerner, R.M., & Korn, S.J. (1972). The development of body-build stereotypes in males. *Child Development,* **43**, 908-920.

Lerner, R.M., & Schroeder, C. (1971). Physique identification, preference, and aversion in kindergarten children. *Developmental Psychology,* **5**, 538.

Richardson, S.A., Goodman, N., Hastorf, A.H., & Dornbusch, S.M. (1961). Cultural uniformity in reaction to physical disabilities. *American Sociological Review,* **26**, 241-247.

Sheehan, G. (1986). Never sell your body short. *American Health,* **5**(6), 100.

Staffieri, J.R. (1967). A study of social stereotype of body image in children. *Journal of Personality and Social Psychology,* **7**, 101-104.

Stout, C., Morrow, J., Brandt, E.N., Jr., & Wolf, S. (1964). Unusually low incidence of death from myocardial infarction: Study of an Italian-American community in Pennsylvania. *Journal of the American Medical Association,* **188**, 845-849.

Swenson, E.J., & Conlee, R.K. (1979). Effects of exercise intensity on body composition in adult males. *Journal of Sports Medicine,* **19**, 323-326.

Wooley, O.W., & Wooley, S.C. (1981). Overeating as substance abuse. *Advances in Substance Abuse,* **2**, 41-67.

Wooley, O.W., & Wooley, S.C. (1982). The Beverly Hills eating disorder: The mass marketing of anorexia nervosa. Dept. of Psychiatry, University of Cincinnati Medical School, **1**(3), 57-68.

Wooley, O.W., Wooley, S.C., & Dryenforth, S.R. (1972a). Obesity and women: I. A closer look at the facts. *Women's Studies International Quarterly,* **2**, 69-77.

Wooley, O.W., Wooley, S.C., & Dryenforth, S.R. (1972b). Obesity and women: II. A neglected feminist topic. *Women's Studies International Quarterly,* **2**, 81-92.

Wooley, S.C., Wooley, O.W., & Dryenforth, S.R. (1979). Theoretical, practical, and social issues in behavioral treatments of obesity. *Journal of Applied Behavior Analysis,* **12**, 3-25.

Zuti, W.B., & Golding, L.A. (1976). Comparing diet and exercise as weight reduction tools. *The Physician and Sportsmedicine,* **4**, 49-53.

Index